GW00645488

HOW TO TAKE 10 YEARS
OFF YOUR FACE
WITHOUT SURGERY

AND ADD
10 YEARS TO YOUR LIFE
NATURALLY

Barbara Frank

Holistic **Health Pra**ctitioner

Acknowledgements to Rick Long, Walter Watson, Jesse Studymeyer, Bonnie Miller, John Alexander, Patricia Shakesphere, Arnold Sawislak, Bill Edwards, Fred Llewellyn, Stuart Eisenberg, Gladys Clearwaters, M. Stansel, Mr. Blalock and Martin Windsor.

All rights reserved. No part of this publication may be reproduced, retitled or reworded, stored in a retrieval system, or transmitted in any form by any means, electronic, mechanical, photocopying, recording, or otherwise, except by the inclusion of brief quotations in a review, without the prior permission in writing from the publisher.

> This book is not intended to replace the services of a physician. It is intended to help nurture and heal the whole person: mind, body and spirit, and prevent debilitating disease. In some cases it can, but it is not intended to provide comprehensive medical information, especially when other or heroic measures are necessary. If you use the information to effect a cure, then you are utilizing your right to self-treatment.

© 1992 by B. Frank

All rights reserved under International and Pan
A M E R I C A N
Copyright Conventions. Published in the United States of America

Library of Congress Catalog Card Number: 94-75253

Manufactured in the United State of America

ISBN 1-884994-00-8

PO Box 5932
Bethesda MD 20824
August 2019
12th Edition

Substantial discount for quantity orders contact jscott2222@hotmail.com

Youth is not a time of life; it is a
  state of mind,
It is not a matter of rosy cheeks,
  red lips and supple knees;
It is a matter of the will,
A quality of the imagination, a
  vigor of the emotions;
It is the freshness of deep springs
  of life.

Samuel Ullman
Ullman, Alabama

This book is for all the ugly ducklings in the world. I was ugly once and the people I thought I loved, my six brothers and sisters, called me "ugly duckling." I thought, as I cried, don't they know their dear sister is in this ugly body, suffering miserably from their cruelty?

Yet if they had not, I would not be here beautiful today!

Lesson From Hinduism

Testimonials

Dear Barbara, thank you for helping me get rid of 5 brain tumors. I am now well. Eternally grateful that you were there when I needed you most. D.

Barbara helped me to see when I was blind. Words cannot express my gratitude. G.

I had COPD and Barbara's treatment was the only thing that healed me. What she knows, all of us need it. V.

I was in Hospice and Barbara helped me to recover and leave with one of her products. I will not be without it. R.

I had ovarian cancer. One session with Barbara, and I healed. It was a God-sent miracle. S.

I had pancreatic cancer third stage. Barbara's protocols helped me to recover. I stared at death's door as the Dr said there was no hope for me. I am the happiest person in the world. T.

I had Lymphatic Cancer, Hodgkins Lymphoma. Barbara's protocols put me in remission and I feel great now. Praise Jehovah! C.

I had Multiple-Myeloma, the Drs gave up on me. Barbara's protocols saved my life. JO

I had breast cancer. Barbara showed me how to heal the cancer without surgery. I am now well. S.

They said I needed a knee replacement. I heard about this woman and sure enough she taught me how to heal my knees and I did not have to have the surgery. Doing well now with no knee pain thanks to Barbara. E.

I was very ill with Lupus. My friend from 20 years before told me I had to see Barbara Frank. After one Lymphatic session with her, I felt restored. I have followed her suggestions and remained well and thanking God every day for her. MM.

I had MS so bad I could not work or focus for the pain it caused. I stayed in bed all the time. A church member told me to go to Barbara. After one Lymphatic Drainage I felt so well I went home and did 8 loads of laundry. Since then I use the Rose cream daily and it seems to be all I need to keep well. Anj.

http://barbarafrank222.com/	*Barbara Frank's website*
https://www.youtube.com/user/darialong3/community	*Barbara Frank videos*
https://darialong.wixsite.com/dlshealthandbeauty	*Barbara's Makeover*
https://www.ebay.com/sch/dlsbeauty/m.html?item=302587791714&hash=item4673a34962%3Am%3AmuyOvb0ftE7Mb_FG1m138sw&rt=nc&_trksid=p2047675.l2562	*Gift Shop*
http://barbarafrank222.com/page1	*The Barbara Frank Show*
https://www.realtruthuniverse.com/archives-2017	*3 Years of Barbara Frank on this show*

Some versions may need to copy and paste links to their browser.

DEDICATED to my mother, Willie Ruth.

ALSO BY BARBARA FRANK

HOW TO STOP SMOKING TODAY

A SURE THING

My name is Barbara Frank, I'm 69 years old and people say I look 30. Please see my videos on youtube and you can determine that for yourself. The mere fact that I can look young and beautiful at age 69 with beautiful thick hair and flawless skin should make every one of you want to do what I am doing to keep myself in good shape and keep your body vitally healthy.

I am totally willing to share with you everything I know and have learned over the years. I hold nothing back when I consult with people. So I advise you to use what I know to get yourself healthy and kill the parasites that are the plaque of mankind because they cause every disease and often cripple and maim us before they kill us. Here you will find the only comprehensive and effective pure organic protocol that exists to eliminate parasites at a very reasonable cost in what we call The Package. It only takes 5 minutes a day. For assistance, questions (barbara_20815@hotmail.com) or to book a telephone consult, go to: barbarafrank222.com and click on products then follow prompts.

The most important thing you need to get from this book is the secret to eternal health, youth and beauty, and with the book, The Package and/or The Consult, I do my best to give it to you.

Even though I am very much into keeping the body mind and spirit vitally healthy, it was doing DL's makeover that made me look like a star. I hesitated before doing it thinking, I look healthy, that's all that matters, I don't need to look like a star. Then I thought, let's face it, in our society, the better you look, the further you get. Just look at all the movie stars who make millions for one picture. We all deserve that. But only those who feel they deserve it will go after it.

I'm really not trying to be a star, I decided I should be all I can be, so I urge you girls and women who want to be all you can be to do DL's makeover. She knows everything about skin care and makeup, I've actually learned a lot from her. See my before and after pictures. What a difference! I've put a link to her website on my products page just look to the left and it's here.

https://darialong.wixsite.com/dlshealthandbeauty

All statements and product recomendations in this book have not been evaluated by the US Food and Drug Administration. These products are not intended to diagnose, treat, cure, or prevent any disease. Anyone using the information here does so at their own risk. The author assumes no responsibility or liability.

CONTENTS

PART 1
HOW TO TAKE 10 YEARS OFF YOUR FACE NATURALLY

I   A Sure Thing I

1   It Happened To Me-
It Can Happen To You! 3

2   This Incredible Information
Can Change Your Life Remarkably 7

3   Using Retin-A Safely 10

4   Recommended Dosage of Retin-A 31

5   You Can Reverse The Ravages of Age 35

6   How To Re-Shape Your Face To Be More Attractive 40

7   How To Change The Contours Of Your Face 47

8   How To Get An Instant Face Lift 50

9   How To Use Retin-A To Make Your Back,
Thighs And Buttocks Beautiful 52

10   How To Get Rid of Dark Circles Under The Eyes 54

11   What Makes Those Ugly Wrinkles, Anyway? 56

12   Some Other Things That Cause Wrinkles 58

13   Learn Something From Babies 60

CONTENTS

PART 2
HOW TO ADD 10 YEARS TO YOUR LIFE NATURALLY

14   First Things First 64

15   There Are Some Good Bacteria 88

16   Did We Really Do All That Damage To Our Planet? 96

17   What We Can Do To Protect Ourselves 103

18   Heal The Body Naturally With Homeopathy 131

19   About Oxygen, The Most Healing Substance On Earth 146

20   Even People Who Have Been
      Health Conscious All Their Lives Benefit From Oxygen 158

21   Fighting Cancer And AIDS With Oxygen, Homeopathy And Minerals, A Cure In Most
      Cases 166

22   101 Ways To Heal The Body Naturally 184

23   Now Anyone Can Lose Weight
      And Keep It Off, For Life 203

24   Keeping Toned For Life 212

25   Mind And Body, Are They One? 218

26   Awareness, The Difference That
      Makes All The Difference 225

27   Heal The Heart, Feed The Soul 240

28   The Most Important Things
      I Do That Keep Me Young 246

29   How To Eliminate The Pain That Millions
      Suffer In Silence 248

30   A Natural Cure For Impotence
      And Menstrual Problems 252

31   A Natural Cure For Migraine Or Any Headache 259

32   Grants, Scholarships And Co-Op Education
      Could Make Your Dreams Come True 263

PART 1

HOW TO TAKE 10 YEARS OFF YOUR FACE WITHOUT SURGERY NATURALLY

Chapter 1

IT HAPPENED TO ME- IT CAN HAPPEN TO YOU!

There is something indescribably delicious about being beautiful!! I want to be beautiful absolutely as long as I live, and I plan to! Sometimes it feels like being one of those 100-foot tall balloons in the Macy's Thanksgiving Day Parade. You feel as if you are spread out over the town for everyone to see, because some people look so intensely.

For more than thirty years I lived on this earth as a plain woman. Then I was transformed into a beautiful woman by the processes I am going to describe to you. *There is a tremendous difference between being plain-looking and being beautiful!* People in America not only <u>respect</u> beauty, they worship it!

Since I have been beautiful all kinds of wonderful things happen to me that never happened when I was blah. I get treated like a celebrity and get all kinds of concessions just because I am beautiful. I receive adoration, gifts, freebies, dinners and invitations from gorgeous, intelligent, successful men and women.

Freud was right when he said "Anatomy is destiny." Having a beautiful anatomy is the easiest way to ensure that you will attract friends and lovers and have a wonderful life. Think about this, have you ever seen an ugly movie star? And of all the rock stars out there, what percentage of them are attractive? Look at the people you see on television; almost all of them are beautiful. You won't find a lot of pockmarked faces and double chins.

Watching all these beautiful people as we do on television day after day, year after year leads to what is known as the **Demonstration Effect** (that which is demonstrated as normal in the many episodes we watch becomes what we expect normal to be).

We feel abnormal when we don't live up to the demonstrated standard, which does not include acne scars, pudgy stomachs and wrinkles. If you have not noticed this consciously before and have lived with it as an almost subliminal phenomenon, please take this opportunity to observe it on the conscious level.

Since we will never be able to change this standard, our options are: conform to it, or pretend it doesn't exist and that we are not affected by it, or simply and realistically try to make the most of living with it.

You can say all this emphasis on beauty is superficial, but the record speaks for itself. We spend 40 billion dollars a year to make ourselves more attractive, and 24 billion dollars on weight-loss products.[1]

Beauty is "in." It always has been and always will be.

Besides, it is fun to be beautiful. Why settle for fourth or fifth place when you can be number one and getting all you can out of life? I never let any of the fuss go to my head. In fact, most of my friends are old ones, and the people who make all these concessions for me are only acquaintances and associates, but I wouldn't go back to looking plain for anything! And there is a difference with my old friends. I think it is respect!

Now no one has to settle for ugly skin, pimples or wrinkles, which, whether you want to admit it or not, have a tremendous effect on your life! People automatically put us into a category according to our appearance, social status, age group and economic status.

There is another aspect of the Demonstration Effect that is more upsetting-everyday hundreds of incidents of justifiable homicide are demonstrated convincingly on television. We cheer when the hero destroys the villain. Nothing proves it more than the show where a child is raped and the mother, while temporarily insane, shoots the rapist in the courtroom after he is declared not guilty. All the people watching cheered as the rapist fell, mortally wounded.

Our children grow up with these shows as their baby-sitters. Is there any wonder that there are so many homicides? The message they get is clearly that if someone does something unforgivable to you, then they deserve to bite the dust, which is usually in a violent manner. Just look at other countries that don't have so much violent TV programming as we do. Their homicide rates are low compared to ours.

---

[1] Micro Diet, 2440 Impala Drive, Carlsbad, CA 92008

As a first grade teacher I saw young boys hurl themselves at each other in fits of anger that I felt was behavior they had learned from some influence, and at first I thought it was their parents. But after meeting them, I knew I had to find another cause, and I did not have to look far.

Most cartoons have characters doing each other in with violence. All you have to do is watch a super heros cartoon, any cartoon, to see the unmitigated violence. Kids are so impressionable, how can we blame them when they grow up and kill each other when this kind of behavior is a big part of their education from such an early age? It used to be that church had a balancing effect, but with the deterioration of the family, the numbers of families and individuals going to church declined.

I know people who live their lives as if what goes on on TV is reality. They take the soaps seriously. Watching and admiring soaps makes them pattern their lives after them, which means they are trying to emulate a series of frustrating incidents. Shit is always happening in the soaps. If that's what I have to do to keep from being boring or bored, I'd rather be boring.

The birth of my first child changed me, for it started me on the road to health. I started spending hours in the health section of the library, with her along, of course. I had always been concerned with my health and exercised and ate moderately well, but I became bent on getting the best of everything for this precious, tiny creature. That quest, which was to create an emotionally and physically healthy, balanced environment where her life could be lived with love, zest and richness, ultimately led to this book.

When I read a scientific study which concluded that babies that were massaged five minutes a day grew twice as large and twice as *smart* as those that were not, I became curious about massage. That article drew me into holistic healing.

Holistic healing encompasses healing the mind, body and spirit using natural remedies or tried and true homeopathic remedies, which are always natural. Holistic healing assumes that all illness involves a degree of imbalance between mind, body and spirit and that all modalities of healing, ancient or new, should be considered.

This book can help you become one of the elite few who enjoy longevity, above-average health, vitality and a youthful appearance, even in your advanced years! Many of us have things in common, some of which include, peace of mind, the ability to effectively run our brains, instead of vice versa, an exercise program, a good diet, healthy relationships and emotional and spiritual peace. It can also save you thousands of dollars in medical expenses and help you protect yourself from some common devastating illnesses like cancer, AIDS, arteriosclerosis, high blood pressure, high cholesterol, migraine, impotence, senility and too many others to name.

Included are many mind-opening bits of information that will change your life dramatically for the better. In the end, you will understand better how important all the information is.

It was only from researching and growing that I realized how unlimited my potential was in any area I chose, particularly keeping my robustly healthy and youthful appearance. I came to realize that I could have tremendous power over my appearance, health and life, and that I could also accelerate my evolving and dynamite away my limitations. Who wouldn't go for all that if presented with the opportunity?

Do you miss being young or attractive? I can show you how to change your appearance if age has crept up on you and wrinkles, ugly skin, pimples, skin discolorations, acne scars, slack facial skin, age and liver spots are preventing you from being beautiful in a world where beauty is of paramount importance. If you are overweight, you can lose weight without being hungry. If mental or emotional "junk" is bogging you down, there is help for that too.

After reading this book you should experience a higher level of consciousness. One of the most important reasons for this book is because I get tired of seeing needless illness and death from chronic diseases that should never have occurred in the first place if nature had not been interfered with. If we stop processing our food to death we have a better chance to get the nutrients that nature intended for us to get from it. The health talk presented can help add ten years and much depth to your existence because you will become aware of numerous life-giving as well as life-threatening hazards that you were not aware of, many of which could profoundly affect you and your family's life and health.

Chapter 2

> # THIS INCREDIBLE INFORMATION CAN CHANGE YOUR LIFE REMARKABLY!

I am close to fifty and yet I look twenty. Though I have maintained my youthful appearance in a variety of ways, like with exercise and diet, the predominant reason for my appearance comes from using Retin-A[2] for the past thirteen years. During that time, I tested different ways to use it and learned incredible things that can be done with it and some other exfoliants containing alpha hydroxy acids (AHA's) from fruits and vegetables that I will describe later.

The mass media have raved about Retin-A's remarkable ability to remove wrinkles, liver and age spots, acne and acne scars. According to a headline about Retin-A in the Washington Post on January 22, 1988:

Wrinkle Cream Lessens Sun-Caused Damage -- It also stated:

"Fulfilling the ancient dream of preserving youthful skin, scientists reported yesterday that a relatively cheap drug used to treat acne can reverse wrinkles and the other signs of aging caused by the sun."[3]

Another headline in The Washington Post on Retin-A in December, 1988 read:

---

[2] Do not use Retin-A or any exfoliant if you are pregnant or thinking about getting pregnant.

[3] © 1988 by The Washington Post, Washington, DC. Reprinted with permission. By Michael Specter.

Acne Drug Side Effect: New Age in Skin Care?

Wrinkles, Sun Damage Reversed

By Michael Specter
Washington Post Staff Writer

Fulfilling the ancient dream of preserving youthful skin, scientists reported yesterday that a relatively cheap drug used to treat acne can reverse wrinkles and the other signs of aging caused by the sun.

The treatment, using a topical cream called tretinoin, softened rough skin, faded age spots and enriched the complexions of almost every patient who tried it, according to a paper published in today's issue of The Journal of the American Medical Association.

"The article suggests that a new age has dawned," wrote Dr. Barbara A. Gilchrest, of the Boston University School of Medicine, in an accompanying editorial. "An enthusiastic reception for this report is assured."

Dermatologists have for some time suspected that Retin-A, the drug's trade name, helps erase wrinkles caused by the sun. And many have prescribed it for that purpose. But today's report is the first to provide persuasive scientific evidence in support of those claims.

"The effects were far more dramatic than anything I had anticipated," said Dr. John J. Voorhees, chairman of the dermatology department at the University of Michigan Medical School and the chief investigator in the study. "Obviously, the implications are pretty big."

The cosmetics industry long ago turned Ponce de Leon's dream of attaining eternal youth into a billion-dollar industry. But while generations of cosmetic adventurers have tried to reverse the aging process, none has succeeded.

In the Voorhees study, 30 patients ranging in age from 35 to 70 rubbed Retin-A on one forearm daily and

See WRINKLES, A4, Col. 1

A4 FRIDAY, JANUARY 22, 1988

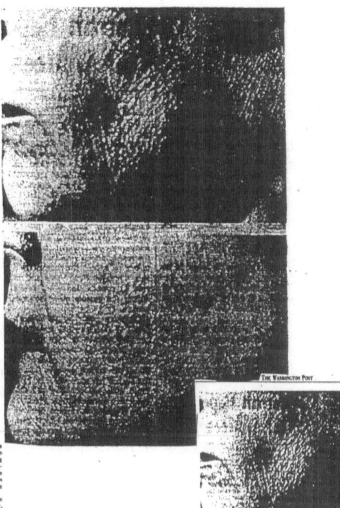

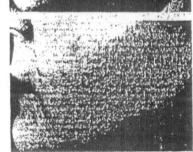

THE WASHINGTON POST

One participant's face was quite wrinkled, above. Tretinoin erased most lines.

UNITED PRESS INTERNATIONAL

Wrinkle Cream Lessens Sun-Caused Skin Damage

WRINKLES, From A1

a cream containing no medication on the other. Half the subjects also tested the drug on their faces. None of them knew which cream contained the drug.

Every patient showed significant reversal of skin damage caused by the sun on the tretinoin-treated forearms but not on the others, according to the report. In addition, all but one of the patients who rubbed tretinoin on their face showed improvement there while none of the others did.

More than 90 percent of the patients experienced temporary inflammation of the skin. "It usually goes away if you stop the drug for a day or two," Voorhees said. "But it's very important to note that this study was done under controlled conditions using high concentrations of cream."

Voorhees said anybody who wants to use the drug should first consult a dermatologist.

Although the study lasted for 16 weeks, Voorhees said yesterday that many of the patients have continued to use the drug for more than a year.

The research was designed to look at the effects of sun on the skin, the cause of nearly all wrinkling, but the scientists also found that the treatment appeared to improve wrinkles caused solely by aging as well.

The researchers found that 30 percent of tretinoin-treated forearms showed slight improvement, 40 percent showed definite improvement and 30 percent showed great improvement.

There is no way of knowing whether continued use after the initial four months will have an improved clinical effect. Voorhees said he has had trouble getting volunteers to stop using the drug so can make comparisons.

Because dermatologists have used tretinoin for more than years in treating acne, its side effects have been studied extensively. In the Michigan trial, skin problems caused by the drug lasted two weeks to three months, according to the report. Forty patients entered the study. Three left because of severe inflammation and seven for personal reasons unrelated to the treatment.

Retin-A is technically available only for treating acne. Its maker, Ortho Pharmaceutical Corp., which paid for part of the Michigan study, is seeking approval to market it for wider use. A 20-gram tube of the cream costs about $20 at most Washington-area pharmacies. And doctors said yesterday that amount could last at least two months.

Once a drug is approved by the Food and Drug Administration for one use doctors are free to prescribe it in other ways as well. Many dermatologists have already begun giving their patients the drug for sun-damaged skin.

"Many of my patients are aware of it. And I have prescribed the drug for wrinkles," said Dr. Philip G. Prioleau, director of dermatologic surgery at New York Hospital-Cornell Medical Center. "For acne it has proven extremely effective. It could even turn out to help prevent skin cancer caused by the sun," he added.

The Michigan group also found tentative evidence that the drug improved premalignant cells in the skin.

Use of the drug has been shown to produce a wide variety of metabolic changes within skin cells, causing them to multiply faster and

to manufacture proteins in different proportions.

The outer layer of the skin, called the epidermis, becomes thinner as it ages or is damaged by the sun. That causes fine wrinkles just below the surface where blood vessels supplying the skin have been reduced in number over time.

As the aging process intensifies, collagen, which maintains the shape and elasticity of the skin, also diminishes.

Tretinoin stimulates the collagen and nearly triples the thickness of the epidermis. That makes the skin stronger and more wrinkle resistant.

© 1988 by The Washington Post, Washington, D.C. Reprinted with permission. By Robin Henig.

Wrinkle Cream: More Promising Findings It further stated:

"Voorhees reported that the signs of "photo-aging"-fine wrinkles, liver spots, splotchiness and sagging skin-cleared up "significantly" more after 10 months than they had after four months, and the improvement was maintained for 12 months after that."[4]

Yet whenever I have spoken to anyone who used Retin-A according to the manufacturer's instructions, they said that it was terrible. It wrinkled their skin, it made them peel, it burned. Yet I have never had any of these results, mainly because I discovered early on that there is a secret to using Retin-A.

Be aware that there are products with names that sound similar, one of which is Retinol, which does not contain tretonin, the active ingredient in Retin-A, and thus, can not give you the exfoliation you need. It does contain 100,000 I.U. of vitamin A, which is good for the skin.

Retin-A is a product that is made from vitamin A, which was originally used to treat acne. Its trade name is tretonin. It must be prescribed by a doctor and there has not been an occasion that I know of where one of my clients called his doctor using the script below and got turned down for a prescription. There are other exfoliants that you can use if you choose not to use Retin-A.

Some people have argued with me that their doctor would never give them a prescription, yet when they called the doctors always did. You simply call your doctor and say, "Hey, I've been reading all the pros and cons about this stuff, Retin-A, and after weighing them, I decided I need a large tube of the cream, .05 percent. I want to try it. I take full responsibility for using it. Here is my pharmacy number. And make it refillable, please."

Remember, your doctor works for you, and whether you have been seeing him for years, or even only a few months, he should have no problem calling in the prescription for you. At the time that I started using Retin-A thirteen years ago, a tube cost 9 dollars. It now commands about 30 dollars for the same size tube, so you see what demand has done to cost, but a tube should last a year. If used correctly, it could last two to four years. What a lot you will be getting for

---

[4] © 1988 by The Washington Post, Washington, D.C. Reprinted with permission. By Robin Henig.

your money! Make sure you take a picture of yourself before you begin this treatment because the change will be very conspicuous.

Still having doubts? Following is a headline from the New York Times about Retin-A:

STUDY FINDS CREAM CLEARS AGE SPOTS

"Doctors who tested the cream found that it lightened or cleared up the age spots in more than 80 percent of users."[5]

The following is reprinted with permission of Hippocrates/ Health Magazine, 310 Howard Street, San Francisco, CA 94105 Jan./Feb. 1988.

DRUGS

No More Wrinkles?   ANN GIUDICI FETTNER

With Retin-A, a cream long prescribed for acne, I have eliminated years of the sun's damage.

I'D COME TO FEEL like the victim of a cruel joke, with a lined, old face capriciously stuck atop a still-young body. But the high cost of having spent the first half of my life sunning thin, fair skin was a cobweb of lines that simply spelled age. I no longer looked like "me," and the worst part of it was knowing that it wasn't going anywhere but downhill.

Then my sister sent me a birthday present, a small tube of a prescription cream called Retin-A, made by the Ortho Pharmaceutical Corporation. "I got us both one," she said. "It's that vitamin A cream that's made Sally look so wonderful. Let's give it a shot."

Hard to believe, but ten to 15 years of age have disappeared. No, there aren't

any before-and-after pictures, because I didn't think it would work, either. But after four months, the lines fanning from my lower lip across my chin have perceptibly faded. The little scrub-boards around my eyes are barely palpable, and my normally sallow skin now has an apricot hue. Even the sagging places under my eyes and along my lower jaw seem diminished. Retin-A will never be able to smooth out the deeper crevices, and I can't go sunbathing anymore because the drug makes my skin burn too easily. But who'd trade this new lease on looks for a tan? People I haven't seen for a while say, "You've done something." I sure have — I've eliminated years of damage caused by the sun with a cream that until recently was used only for acne.

Like many discoveries, that of Retin-A's ability to reverse the sun's damage was serendipitous. In the late 1960s, dermatologist Albert M. Kligman of the University of Pennsylvania developed an acne medication called tretinoin, a synthetic derivative of vitamin A and the active

ingredient in Retin-A. Though most of the people using the drug were young, Kligman began to hear comments that the cream seemed to make their skin smoother. After several years of such reports, he decided to see if and how such changes were really occurring.

In 1983, Kligman and his co-workers set up an experiment in which eight people, aged 68 to 77, used the tretinoin cream on their faces for six to 12 months; six women used a similar cream that lacked the drug. In addition, 15 women used Retin-A cream on one forearm and the placebo cream on the other. The study was small, but Kligman says the improvement in the treated skin was indisputable.

Under the microscope, a biopsy of 50-year-old facial skin reveals extensive

[5] © 1992 by The New York Times Company. Reprinted by permission.

damage, most caused by the sun. The epidermis, the skin's top layer, is thickened and littered with dead cells. Pigmented cells collect in the bottom of the epidermis, causing brown "liver spots." Beneath, the formerly elastic layer called the dermis now has few collagen fibers — the protein that gives skin its structure. Cell production is lethargic; sun-damaged skin takes twice as long as normal skin to create new cells and push them up to the epidermis. The cells are different sizes and shapes, sometimes clumped together; the result is a scaly, wrinkled look.

Enter Retin-A. After a couple of nights of washing with a mild soap, drying thoroughly, and applying Retin-A, my face began to look and feel sunburned. It was working! In about ten days the rawness faded, and a layer of skin rubbed off when I smoothed on a moisturizing cream. Underneath was a glossy shine I hadn't seen in decades.

Here's what is happening, according to Kligman's preliminary studies: Retin-A seems to thin the epidermis and to step up cell production. The quickly multiplying new cells push the dead cells off the skin's surface more rapidly. That's the shine I've noticed — fresh, plump cells. New blood vessels also form, and the increased flow of blood makes the skin look rosy. Some preliminary studies even suggest that new collagen fibers begin to crisscross the dermis, restoring a youthful firmness. It all adds up to smoother, glowing skin that seems to have fewer fine wrinkles.

Lest you get carried away, however, there are drawbacks. "For certain people, the change is only slight," says dermatologist Arthur K. Balin of the Rockefeller University, who has even prescribed Retin-A for his mother. Some can't use the cream because it irritates their faces too much, he says. In addition, because the drug thins the epidermis and leaves fewer dead cells to protect it, the skin is more prone to sunburn and further damage from the sun. "But it's certainly the only cream available," says Balin, "that actually does something for wrinkles."

And is Retin-A safe? It's a good question, and for the moment it's not settled, although physicians don't seem worried.

In mice, the combination of Retin-A and artificial sunlight has apparently speeded the development of skin tumors. However, other research shows that

Retin-A reverses tumors. In addition, the class of chemicals that includes tretinoin has actually been used to treat some skin cancers as well early cervical cancer.

In fact, Ortho Pharmaceutical is currently sponsoring studies that so far indicate the drug reverses certain precancerous skin conditions. And there's apparently no increase in cancer among the thousands of acne patients who have used Retin-A for the last 16 years. "I'm not worried," says Samuel Stegman, former president of the American Society for Dermatologic Surgery. "We're using very low doses. And the mice that developed tumors were exposed to sunlight — but people using the cream have been warned about the damage the sun can do, and they know to stay out of the sun."

Given all this, you'd think that Retin-A would have seriously shaken up the $543-million-a-year market for facial lotions and moisturizers. But getting Retin-A requires a trip to the doctor for a prescription. And it's currently approved by the Food and Drug Administration for use as an acne treatment only. This doesn't mean it's illegal to use for sun-damaged skin: A doctor can prescribe a drug for any purpose once it's approved for some use. But it does mean that Retin-A's safety and effectiveness as an "anti-aging" cream haven't been proven — Kligman's studies and anecdotal reports are the only evidence so far — and that Ortho can't advertise it as such. That could change: Depending on the outcome of the tests Ortho is funding, the company intends to ask the FDA to approve Retin-A as a treatment for sun damage and for precancerous lesions.

Retin-A isn't the only threat to the anti-wrinkle-cream industry. Several other products are in the works, such as DHEA

(dehydroepiandrosterone), a naturally occurring hormone that restores oil production and may rebuild collagen, blood vessels, and skin cells. Developed by dermatologist Norman Orentreich of New York University, it has yet to be submitted for FDA approval. Harvey Miller of Daltex Medical Sciences in West Orange, New Jersey, has filed a patent for a chemical related to Retin-A that is taken as a pill. And a mysterious substance called Factor X, created by the British biotechnology company Senetek, is about to be tested in Europe.

Cosmetic companies won't comment on any of these products. This may be because of the industry's problems with its own "anti-aging" creams. Their recent ads claiming that some skin care products promote "cellular repair" and other biological changes has prompted the FDA to send letters to 23 companies saying that such statements qualify the products as drugs — and that the companies must either stop making the claims or apply for approval of the cosmetics as drugs.

If you want to be completely on the safe side, you should wait until Retin-A (or any drug, for that matter) has been thoroughly tested. But if you opt for Retin-A now, make sure to use it under a doctor's supervision.

Dermatologists suggest using the cream every night for a year to 18 months and only on weekends after that. They caution that not everyone sees dramatic changes and that Retin-A can't eliminate the deeper wrinkles. For instance, my dark-skinned sister isn't experiencing nearly the effects that I am. Thin-skinned Celtic types, who suffer more damage to begin with, seem to benefit more. Retin-A can be very irritating, so use a moisturizer. In addition, it's very important to use a sunscreen every day: After the one day I walked around unprotected, my face looked and felt scalded. Retin-A costs about $20 for a three-months' supply.

I figure that's a bargain. Underneath its new surface, my skin is microscopically changing appearance from that of a long-abandoned wall with the stones kicked down and scattered to one whose layers are dense and neatly arranged. My proof? When your 14-year-old, who hasn't really looked at you in years, says, "Ma, you're looking great!" you know something more than wishful thinking is going on. ▣

Chapter 3

USING RETIN-A SAFELY

Before you begin this therapy test your reaction to Retin-A by doing the traditional patch test by applying it inside your arm for five days before you start using it. If you normally just brush over this area when you shower because it rarely gets dirty anyway, pay special attention and wash it everyday during the test week. Use a small amount, the smallest amount possible, the same amount that you are going to use on your face. It should appear transparent on your finger.

To get the right dose, barely touch your finger to the cream. It is very concentrated. Rub Retin-A in for one or two minutes every night for five nights. Check your arm everyday for a week, and if there are no ill effects you may begin treatment on the sixth night.

If there is too much inflammation, irritation or discoloration from using Retin-A, you may want to try the milder exfoliants. They are made from fruit and vegetable acids and listed under Moisturizers below. If you experience too much irritation from using any product, do not use it. Too much irritation is excessive peeling, irritation, discoloration or blistering of the skin.

Two minutes after applying moisturizer, apply the smallest amount of Retin-A possible to cover the size of a pencil eraser head by dotting it on your forehead, cheeks and chin and rubbing it in. I mean the amount you use should be minuscule, for Retin-A is a powerful exfoliator.

If your skin is not especially fragile and you had no bad reaction from the patch test, massage Retin-A in for about one minute. If your skin is oily and pimply, gradually work up to massaging Retin-A in for about three minutes two or three times a week. Rub your skin in the direction you would like it to stay in. For example, never pull down on your skin. When massaging your face or applying exfoliator, apply by using slow, long horizontal strokes.

Moisturize a minute or so later. Make it a rule to moisturize your skin twice. The second moisturization should occur a minute or so after the first.

Make sure you never go in your bed after being outside without at least washing your exposed skin with warm soapy water. Our air has a lot of microbes and impurities in it and if you go in your bed after outside exposure, you put these impurities in your bed. You need to gently scrub your skin to exfoliate dead skin cells. I can't believe how many people I have met who told me they just stood under the shower and let the water run over their skin for a shower. I was shocked. They were all men.

You will never get clean that way. Also dead skin cells build up and your body develops a stale smell that you become immune to. Like having chronic bad breath. No one wants to tell you your breath is bad, but a real friend should. After bath it is best to apply Rose Beauty Cream undiluted all over the body from face to toes. However for the first month when you start to use Rose Beauty Cream you should dilute it as the instructions recommend. After your body acclimates to it, you will get best results by using it full strength and it will be your armor of protection.

Retin-A comes in various strengths and cream and gel form, the cream being superior. Potencies: 0.025 percent is the weakest, but probably the one you want to start with unless you have used exfoliants in the past; 0.05 percent in cream form is the recommended strength, and 0.01 percent in the red tube is the strongest. You should use the red strength only for thighs and severely damaged skin.

The strength you want to aspire to use for your face is .05 percent in cream form. You may have to start with a weaker strength of Retin-A or an alpha hydroxy acid. Even for the worst acne, start with either the weakest or the middle strength.

Normal skins should start with the weakest strength, and work up to 0.05 percent. I have used the stronger strength on my thighs to remove heavy duty scarring like some of the brutal ones from childhood and from poison ivy. I have never used 0.01 percent on my face and only recommend it for severe acne or severe wrinkling or scarring.

If you went out and had your face lifted (the treatment you are going to learn about is superior to face-lifts, and there is no painful surgery or scaring, in fact, no one needs to know you are using exfoliants except you), you would pay all that money and after a few years you would need to have it done again. With this process you can learn how to control how fast or how slowly you want to peel off your unattractive surface skin. Waiting underneath is a new, younger skin.

Once you peel your old skin away you peel away the years, the wrinkles, the splotches, the age spots - - and you don't have to allow them to come back! That is the power that exfoliating gives you!

The Most Important Rule

Let your skin be the judge of how often you use exfoliants. In the beginning use exfoliant every third night, then more often if your skin allows. With alpha hydroxy acids sometimes if you use them for three consecutive days and nights they become too harsh and you may have to stay off of them for a few days.

If the peeling or irritation is too severe, stop until it completely clears up. You may only need to use an exfoliant once a month, depending on your skin's reaction to it. Do not continue to use exfoliant if you experience too severe irritation. You should be able to regulate your dosage to the point that the skin exfoliates invisibly and without severe irritation, be that everyday or once a month.

If your skin becomes too sensitive, skip exfoliants for a few days or a week. During that time continue to wash or cleanse to help get the exfoliating skin off. Remember, if you don't it can become impacted. You can hide the fact that you are giving yourself a new skin by waiting one minute after you wash your face and using *Curel*. This renders your exfoliating skin invisible and effectively hides it.

In some cases a kind of porosity may appear during the first few weeks that you use Retin-A. I realized that it is so subtle no one notices me closely enough to notice it, and it goes away as that layer of skin is removed. The end results are worth suffering a few days of over-porosity. Porosity can be minimized by using Cetaphil and/or Sea Breeze for the skin. If the over-porosity bothers you, use a tad (same dosage as Retin-A), of cortisone cream at night once in a while.

```
┌─────────────────────────────────┐
│                                 │
│      Important To Remember      │
│        About The Face           │
│                                 │
└─────────────────────────────────┘
```

Do not scrub your skin deeply and vigorously with the hope of speeding up the exfoliating process. Continue to wash as you always have. I wash my face with a wash cloth in a circular motion while pushing up on my skin.

After you have used exfoliants for years you will be able to scrub with the exfoliating-type of facial sponges that have come on the market recently, but that will be because you will have constructed yourself an entirely new complexion by then. Using an abrasive during the early stages will just damage and discolor your fragile, new skin.

Allow your skin to fall off and peel off naturally. If you follow these instructions for using exfoliants, you will barely be able to notice yourself that your skin is peeling off, and that is how it should be. In the past, women have gone nuts and discontinued Retin-A because the peeling from it made them look too unsightly.

They used it incorrectly and the results they got were unfavorable. They did not benefit from this miraculous discovery because they did not use it properly. The only time you will see your skin exfoliating is when you are not following my instructions!

As much as you will probably be tempted, do not force or coerce your skin to peel. Your new skin will be very sensitive to the sun, so keep your face out of the sun for long periods of time.

Since sunshine is very healing, necessary for metabolic processes and essential to good health, don't avoid the sun. It is true that sun can cause skin cancer, so it must be taken in moderation. It has too many advantages to avoid it. It has been found to destroy parasites, viruses and disease in the body, and stimulate libido.

I encourage you to get sunshine on your body. You can get sun on your body without getting it on your face. However, you do need to get a few minutes a day of direct sunlight on your eyes. It is not necessary to look directly at the sun in order to do this. It is advised that you do not look directly at the sun. Allow it to shine into your eyes.

It stimulates the pineal gland, which is called the anti-aging gland. If you go in the sun for extended periods of time, wear sunscreen and a hat. If you notice warts or moles starting to appear on your skin, this means that you are getting too much sun. Tests showed that Retin-A eliminated pre-cancerous lesions on the skin. It is even used now to prevent cervical cancer. Check with your doctor before trying it this way.

If you want to test Retin-A and just use it on one undesirable spot, try using it on just that area, for certainly the inner arm and the facial complexion are two different types of skin. You will have an opportunity to compare the new skin that emerges from the use of Retin-A to the old skin you had all along. Then you can decide which skin you prefer to live with.

> ## Watch Your Skin For Discolorations!

Remember, KEEP A CLOSE CHECK ON THIS! If your skin starts to darken in places, particularly in the places where new skin is appearing, then start using a small amount of my natural herbal Southern Rose cream to eliminate discolorations.

DISCOLORATION means two things: *1. That you are either scrubbing too hard and peeling off the new skin before it is time, or 2. That you probably need to wash less frequently and gentler. You probably need to cleanse with Cetaphil as an alternative to soap and water. Remember,* this may also mean you will not need to use exfoliant nightly, only about three times a week. Let your skin be your guide. Once a week may be enough for you. You will understand this better as you continue to use exfoliants.

> ## Moisturizers

It used to be that we all had nothing to look forward to as we grew older but leathery-looking skin and masses of wrinkles. This fact is no longer so, and one of the reasons is the new breed of moisturizers that have evolved as a result of women's insistence that they must look young and beautiful at any cost and at any age. In the last few years, moisturizers have arrived that are far superior to what we have used traditionally, and these are the ones with alpha-hydroxy acids from fruits, milk, sugarcane, vegetables like beets, cucumbers, corn and synthetic sources. They not only protect skin from harmful sun rays, they also reverse years of sun damage, acne, scarring and wrinkles.

They actually protect your skin from environmental damage like sun which wrinkles and wind which drys and chaps. This is a definite advantage of AHAs over Retin-A, for if you go in the sun while using it, you need to use a good sun block. SPF 15 is recommended. Still, you do not want to spend eight hours in the sun and expect an alpha-hydroxy acid to protect you. Moderation is recommended.

The alpha-hydroxy acids work by ungluing dead skin which sloughs off slower and slower as we age, and by penetrating deep into skin to moisturize and plump up skin cells. As skin exfoliates, new collagen is made the same as when using Retin-A. The advantage of the alpha-hydroxy acids is that they smooth fine lines immediately and give a fresh and polished look to skin right away. Within 10 days, the results are dramatic!

Another advantage these acids have over Retin-A is that they are usually milder and cause less irritation. They also take almost three times longer to remove scars and deep wrinkles than Retin-A takes. Many people hate their skin being irritated and peeling, but you never have to worry about it showing if you follow my instruction of moisturizing twice with my natural herbal Southern Rose cream within two minutes after washing your face.

If using alpha-hydroxy acids, they can be reapplied during the day to remoisturize and exfoliate between the times that you wash your face.

Do the patch test before using any of these exfoliating moisturizers. Your skin may react differently to every one of them. In the beginning, use them over a thin film of moisturizer. You can still re-mold and re-shape your face using them as well because the alpha-hydroxy acids make the skin make new collagen, which is necessary for firm, youthful skin. More on this later.

If alpha-hydroxy acids make you exfoliate too fast, try waiting five or ten minutes after washing your face before applying them. If they still cause too severe irritation, try waiting thirty minutes or an hour. The more moist the skin, the better they penetrate. If they are still too strong, mix a small amount of an AHA-containing moisturizer with a small amount of .·my herb.cream as a·. moisturizer and then apply. Monitor your results with each type of application to see which is most suitable for your skin.

The acid-based moisturizers contain anywhere from 2-4 percent acid for the face and 5-15 percent acid for hands and body, and cost from 2 to 100 dollars an ounce. There are such a large variety of them on the market now and they are being reformulated so fast that you need to be responsible for finding out the percentage of acid in the cream you use. I have tested at least twelve, and I like every one of them. They all work and do what they are supposed to do.

Start with a low percentage. Don't even think of using it everyday until you have been using it for at least three months so your skin can acclimate to it. Then you can gradually increase the strength.

Use a stronger strength on legs and thighs, like Avon's Anew for hands and body which has 10 percent glycolic acid. Always use a moisturizer on top of AHAs. You may even want to use two moisturizers. Sometimes I apply Curel, then Neutrogena's night cream. This extra moisturization can make all the difference for some people.

After trying dozens of moisturizers form all over the world, I chose several as my favorites. My all natural herbal Southern Rose cream, hereafter called SRC, beat all others. It is antimicrobial, antibacterial, antiviral, antidepressant, antiscarring, pain-relieving and kills lice, mites and other microorganisms that people pick up. It is safe for children and ·pets. It makes the skin soft and silky for days after a single application.

I use is as a base under everything, and not just on my face, but all over my body. It contains Vitamins C, A and E, and minerals which are very effective at fighting free radicals (which destroy tissue by stealing electrons from proteins which can start cells to mutating, and so are very desirable in a moisturizer. The people who come to me rave about it. Do not use my Aphrodisiac cream on children.

It works well even if diluted. Minute amounts full-strength work best.

Some of the many moisturizers containing alpha-hydroxy acids that I like are, in order of preference: *All You Need* by Prescriptives, *Fruition* by Estee Lauder, *Anew*[2] by Avon, and Clinique's *Turnaround Cream*, which acts similar to Retin-A in that it is a stronger exfoliator. All of these moisturizers are excellent exfoliants. Presently they are only found at better department stores. However, my favorite exfoliants are SRC and Retin-A, because they eliminates problems faster. So for practical purposes, I will say Retin-A or SRC when I mean exfoliant. You may substitute either of the exfoliants recommended after testing it if Retin-A is not suitable for your skin. What may be best is using Retin-A only on serious problems like gigantic pimples and severe eruptions and then after they settle down, using alpha hydroxy acids and SRC at other times. Ideally, it is best to start exfoliating with the mildest exfoliant, then work up to stronger ones.

All You Need uses tiny water-holding spheres and mild acids from lemon and passion fruit for exfoliating. Fruition uses the enzyme protease to break the bond between living and dead cells and sloughs dead cells off.

Turnaround Cream uses salicylic acids in liposomes to give continuous moisturizing and exfoliating. If you use Turnaround Cream, allow your skin to decide how often. If you use it one night, and two days later your skin feels too tight, then you probably need to use it only once or twice a week. Use very sparingly. These creams make skin look terrific, even with the first application.

Do not use three or four of these exfoliants at a time. I recommend you buy them one at a time and finish one before you start another to properly compare them. Fruition or Turnaround Cream can be used under your moisturizer a week or two after you have stopped applying Retin-A.

All You Need is supposed to be a complete exfoliating moisturizer, and it can be, just remember to use it twice. I moisturize twice with it, then spread a thin layer of Curel over it

---

* Their Anew Perfecting Complex For Hand And Body has more exfoliant than the one designed for the face. It is a good idea to use the one for the face if you start using this exfoliant first. Call 1-800-FOR-AVON. If you have used exfoliants in the near past, then you may be able to start with the stronger formula. Test first.

layer of SRC over it about two minutes after putting it on. Generally, make it a rule to use a non-exfoliating moisturizer over each exfoliating moisturizer.

Some ironclad rules for all exfoliants are: wash or cleanse at least twice, preferably three times a day to remove exfoliating skin; moisturize shortly after cleansing. Always moisturize twice. Between the times that you wash your face, moisturize with SRC, your AHA or both. Keep a small bottle filled with SRC in your purse or in your desk to moisturize your face between washings. Once or twice a day will make a big difference.

I use all these exfoliating moisturizers on a short-term basis. You may find that you need to use them less and less. If your skin is in bad shape, you will need to use them more frequently at first, then gradually you can reduce the frequency of use as your skin improves. Remember, your skin peeling means that what you want to get rid of, your undesirable outer skin, is coming off, and what will surface is new baby skin that is moist, unblemished, fresh and healthy looking.

As I said, SRC is one of my favorite all over body moisturizers. I also like *Moisture* (great for hair and skin) by Especially Hair (301 540-8125), *Nutribel* by Lancome, *Neutrogena's Night Cream*, and L'Oreal's *Plentitude Night Renewal Cream*. Then I found a way to make SRC better. I discovered that if I allowed the water to evaporate out of it, what remained was a moisturizer for the skin superior to most I have ever encountered.

To make the SRC more concentrated, simply cover the inside of a clean cosmetic jar with a thin layer of it. Cover with a tissue and allow to stand overnight before replacing the cover. The water will evaporate, causing the cream to be more concentrated, and you will have your super moisturizer. For even more moisturizing power, squeeze vitamin E from gel caps and mix with SRC. I use this concentrated strength over regular SRC. Or you may already have a moisturizer that you like.

SRC is very inexpensive considering the cost of all the others, yet it performs as well as they do. Remember that vitamin E oil straight from the gel cap is a powerful skin preserver before bed. For example, I use concentrated SRC over Fruition or over Turnaround Cream, and even over the 100 dollar an ounce creams. And over all that, vitamin E. All should be applied frugally.

If you use Turnaround Cream, use regular Curel for your first moisturization, and concentrated Curel for your second. Of course you can use your favorite moisturizer.

Some people can use Retin-A or any of the other exfoliants mentioned above for a week straight and then not use them again for a month. Others can use them for a month straight and not feel any ill effects. Ill effects are: too severe peeling of the skin, irritation and overly red skin. Just let your skin tell you how often to use Retin-A. I have gone without using it for six months.

I find that now I cannot use any exfoliant for more than four days straight. My skin may peel silently for weeks or a month afterwards.

Since skin is composed of protein, and shampoo is formulated to cleanse hair which is pure protein, and because soap has a tendency to dry my skin, I discovered that if I cleansed my face and body with an inexpensive protein shampoo, itching and dryness of the skin decreased dramatically. Any generic brand of protein shampoo like the one you find in your supermarket for thirty-two ounces for a dollar and a half will do. You only need a small amount, and it lasts longer than a bar of soap.

If you are thinking that washing your face three times a day (which will take about one minute, and will massively rehydrate your skin) is going to take too much time or be inconvenient, just think of how much time you will save when you no longer have to apply foundation. As you go along, your beautiful new skin will require less and less maintenance and makeup.

Beautiful skin can be had most easily from within as well. Vitamin C greatly increases the production of collagen, one of the key ingredients for healthy-looking skin. Vitamin A is essential for healthy skin and for the production of natural antibodies against disease. It is also used to cure impotence and cancer. In general, making sure you get the proper amount of vitamins, minerals and enzymes will have a big effect on how your skin looks. Stay away from fried and fatty foods and sugar.

Many dermatologists believe that seafood and foods containing iodine bring on acne. You may want to test this theory by discontinuing all iodine-containing foods for six weeks to see if this may be causing your acne. Some iodine-containing foods are: cheese, butter, milk, sour cream, yogurt, tap water, beef liver, turkey, chicken, wheat germ, chips, white bread and most seafood.

Some people have rashes that come from coming in contact with certain metals. Nickel rash is one of the most common. Make sure your jewelry is not made of nickel and limit your exposure to nickel or nickel-containing metals. Don't eat nickel nuts. Don't use fake nails as they have been found to cause rashes. Wear cotton or natural fibers. Some of the fake or man-made fibers cause rashes. Try drinking Dandelion and Echinacea tea to purify your blood and stimulate your immune system.

One of the main components of our immune system is the thymus gland, which is located beneath the breast bone and which secretes 26 or more hormones that control the complex mechanisms of the body. The thymus gland instructs lymphocytes, interferon, interleukin and killer cells to attack cancer cells and foreign matter in the body. Use the acupressure points below to stimulate the pineal gland to re-balance your hormones and relieve acne, pimples and blemishes.

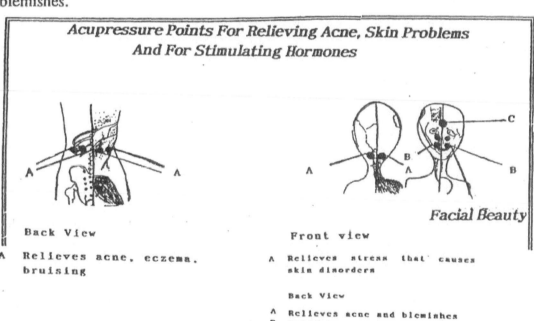

Acupressure Points For Relieving Acne, Skin Problems And For Stimulating Hormones

Facial Beauty

Back View

A   Relieves acne, eczema, bruising

Front view

A   Relieves stress that causes skin disorders

Back View

A   Relieves acne and blemishes
B   Relieves acne, blemishes, sagging cheeks
C   Stimulates the pituitary gland, helps the skin all over body
C   Strengthens immune system, kidneys and adrenal glands. Reduces stress. Induces emotional stability. Balances hormones and the body so acne does not erupt

> ## *If You Have*
> ## *Fragile Skin*

If, after the trial period, there is darkening of the skin, and it looks burned, do not start using exfoliants. Some skins are extremely delicate and can only tolerate minute amounts of exfoliants. Do the patch test again, using a different exfoliant, on the inside of your other arm. Use the moisturizer on your arm one or two minutes before applying the exfoliant. Check your arm everyday. Use the moisturizer and exfoliant on your arm for three days, then monitor for four days more. If no damage is observed, you may begin as instructed.

If you experience slight damage to your skin after the second test (a whitish peeling is normal and will go away when you apply moisturizer), then your skin may be too fragile for exfoliants. To get your skin acclimated to them, use a mild one on your elbows, knees and legs, and allow your body to become accustomed to them.

What happens is as you shower they will be distributed all over your body in minute amounts, and gradually, your skin will adjust to them. Only you can be the judge. I think many people will misinterpret the minor problems (excess peeling or redness, skin too tight) associated with exfoliants and conclude their skin does not adjust to them. Give them a fair chance.

The benefits of using AHAs far outweigh the problems. The benefits are exfoliation of wrinkles and ugly skin to reveal virgin, new skin. The skin begins to make collagen even if it hasn't done this well in years, and facial skin is renewed and improvements are clearly observable. Keep an open mind and watch the beautiful results.

So as you bathe, minute amounts of exfoliant will get into your skin, and you will be able to use it on your face eventually. Just keep testing it under your arm until there is no damage. *Do not use exfoliants on your face if there is damage on the inside of your arm or in any place that you use them. If, after a reasonable amount of time, (1 year) you still experience unreasonable irritation from the test (too severe peeling, discoloration or irritation) then you may be unable to use exfoliants.*

If you know you are one of those people with dry, thin, fragile skin and the skin test did not hurt you, then follow these instructions:

•**Wash your face. Wait one or two minutes. Apply a small amount of moisturizer (SRC or your favorite). Allow to dry (two minutes). Apply a minute amount of exfoliant. Rub in but do not massage. Apply another thin layer of moisturizer. Wait one minute and moisturize again.**

•*If you know you are going to be in the sun the next day do not use Retin-A the night before. If you know you are going to be in the sun for a long period of time and you are currently using Retin-A, wear a hat to protect your face from too much sun exposure. The alpha-hydroxy acids actually protect skin from the sun, but keep in mind that new skin is more fragile, and should be treated as such.*

•*Before sun, follow your usual routine. Apply your AHA and then sunscreen.*

•*Make sure to remember to wash your face three times a day to -allow the exfoliating skin to slough off. Always use a moisturizer after washing. Always moisturize twice.*

After you have been using exfoliant on your face for three months, then you should be able to massage it into your skin for a minute or so when applying it. Remember, whenever you start something new with exfoliants, monitor your results. You will start to learn how to use trial and error to get the results you want.

Sometimes I go for three months without using an exfoliant. Then I get a pimple, or a sunburn, or notice any slight slackening of my skin, and I can use it for three or four days sometimes, and maybe a month later, use it for one or two more days.

This is the point that you will reach as you continue to use exfoliants. Always listen to your skin. If it is crying out, cracking excessively, then you are using far too much exfoliant too often or you are cleansing too harshly. Cut back and try using Cetaphil soapless cleanser some or all of the time instead of soap to wash with. Cetaphil is so convenient that you can keep it in a small bottle in your purse and cleanse your skin anywhere without water. It is also an excellent gentle exfoliant that does no damage and leaves the skin slightly moisturized.

Never use tissues or paper products on your skin as they tear the skin follicle and cause premature wrinkling of the skin. Use a clean cotton cloth to remove the Cetaphil.

> ## What If You Do Not Want
> ## To Wait To Remove
> ## Pimples?!

I've found that you can shorten the life of the huge zits that appear by forcing them out earlier than they had planned to leave. Just soaking a small piece of cotton in regular 3 percent hydrogen peroxide and taping it over the crater. Other things that force them out is vinegar (you may need to dilute it) and the mineral water I sell to my patients. These things can be used as a compress and will force the zit out.

Within two hours, the peroxide will do major damage by dissolving the pus and liquids from the zit. It will actually suck out and destroy the zit, which is a parasite. All pimples are microbes. I have found this to be a highly effective procedure for eliminating zits and getting rid of enormous painful pimples, one at a time. Unfortunately, if you have pimples, you need to use SCR, parts I and II. Instructions are included when you order it. It eliminates the cause of pimples, scarring, wrinkles, cellulite, and causes enormous weight loss. All overweight is caused by microbes. Killing them is the only safe way to lose weight.

> ## *If You Have A Face Full of Pimples - Help Is On The Way*

Recommended for Acne:

Most effective: Southern Rose Cream, Oxygen (pages 151 and 155 in this book),[1] no dairy products or sugar, multiple vitamin and mineral, an egg a day for the sulphur amino acids, a homeopathic combination for acne based on your symptoms. You may also need a homeopathic medicine for infection. See a homeopathic or naturopathic doctor. Take an amino acid supplement. Eat lots of fresh sprouts (properly cleaned, page 80), cooked carrots, take B_6, zinc, 6 glasses of distilled water a day. Use Retin-A or a moisturizer with alpha-hydroxy acids, exercise, meditation, acupressure, drink aloe vera juice, *Kali Bichromicum, Sulphur* (homeopathic).

If your face is full of pimples, you can use either Retin-A or an alpha hydroxy acid-containing moisturizer everyday (if your skin permits) until the severity of your breakouts diminishes. Retin-A is particularly effective at eliminating new breakouts. If you experience uncomfortable drying, drop back on your usage. Pimples microbes being expelled by your body, so think of them as toxins *out*, thank goodness, rather than *inside* you.

To prepare to force them out, find an area where you can use the sun to look at your face with a mirror, preferably a magnifying mirror. Prepare a place where you can soak your face. Just before soaking, wash your face, holding warm, not hot water to the area where the problem is. You are going to be softening the blackheads and whiteheads so that the "ripe" ones can be removed. The warm water will bring a lot of pimples to the surface of your skin. Things that bring them out are: salt, Epsom Salts, peroxide, my Mineral water. Use one or several of the above and soak each side of your face for five to ten minutes.

---

[7] The word was coined by the French chemist Antoine Lavoisier in the 18th century. The French word, oxygene meant acid-producing (from the Greek oxus which means sharp and in the sense of acid, and the Greek suffix genes which means born). At the time oxygen was considered to be an essential part of an acid. Even though this is not true, the name has stuck. In truth, oxygen is a colorless, odorless, tasteless gaseous element that is essential to life and required for combustion.

There are two ways that you can remove them. You can let your skin dry thoroughly (five minutes) and gently use a dry cloth to rub some of them away (only the ones that come out easily). This must be done extremely gently and with a lot of light. This method should cause the least amount of irritation and damage to your skin. You may also apply olive oil and my Southern Rose Cream and massage out the parasites.

After you finish steaming your face, wash it gently with warm water or cleanse with Cetaphil and your favorite moisturizer. Sometimes, at this point, I use ice. It does wonders for the face. After one minute, apply moisturizer. After two minutes apply a small amount of Retin-A (only enough to barely cover the area is more than enough). Retin-A *must* be applied *very* lightly. Remember the warm water will bring a lot of what is in your clogged pores to the surface. After you soak your face you can look at it in the mirror with the sun on it to check this out. At this point you can just wash or cleanse your face again to remove surface oils and debris and allow the pimples to be erased with Retin-A and or my Southern Rose Cream.

With the diet and supplements recommended in this book, the cognitive growth you will experience, the nourishment for your soul, proper exercise and massage to keep your lymph and body fluids flowing smoothly, your acne should disappear. Anyone who says they haven't time for exercise should consider dancing to music in their room. If a person is able to exercise, there simply is no excuse or reason not to when you weigh the value of exercise against the disadvantages of not exercising.

Remember the steam will bring a lot of what is in your clogged pores to the surface. After you steam your face you can look at it in the mirror with the sun on your face to check this out. At this point you can just wash or cleanse your face again to remove surface oils and debris and allow the pimples to be erased with Retin-A and not squeeze anything out.

If you are averse to steaming your face, you can remove pimples by softening them with a cotton cloth soaked in rather warm water. This is not my method of choice since it leaves the skin looking prematurely aged. Retin-A and AHAs can eliminate that later. For example, if you had a face full of pimples and just wanted to get rid of them once and for all and this was the easiest way for you to steam your face, it is okay to use this method for a short while.

•Immediately after washing use Olive Oil, an antiseptic for the skin. After one minute apply SRC. After two minutes apply a small amount of Retin-A (only enough to barely cover the area is more than enough). Retin-A must be applied very lightly.

•To re-close pores, use Revlon Honey Masque mixed with Revlon Egg Masque. Apply after cleansing and moisturizing and leave on for 20-30 minutes. Peel off and look gorgeous.

When you peel the masque off, your skin will be moisturized. Moisturize your skin before doing the masque. At this point, if you moisturize again or do anything to your face, the effect of the masque will quickly go away.

However, if you apply baby powder about five minutes after you take the masque off, let it set for about two minutes then gently brush off, the effect of the masque can last up to two days.

Once you practice these techniques for awhile, you will learn their magic and master them.

Next day monitor your skin to see the effect of the previous day's treatment. If there is no damage, you can use this procedure once a week or bi-weekly.

Taking oxygen, which you will hear more about later, greatly reduced chronic acne. And although Retin-A diminished the acne from without, this diminished it from within.

If you do not have time to steam your face, the best time to remove any pimples is after you come out of the shower.

Removing the deeply embedded whiteheads from your skin will be a gradual but rewarding process. They cause the stale smell that lingers in your pillows and bedclothes.

Removing a pimple may take from two seconds to three minutes depending on the texture of your skin and other factors, but remember, once you remove it, it is gone and you do not have to wait two weeks to a month for it to be over with. Do not spend more than one minute trying to remove a pimple.

Remember also that if you get carried away and tear the skin on your face, you may have to suffer a scar until it disappears. Fortunately Retin-A and SRC can remove the scar, but we do not want to cause any. Retin-A and SRC also decrease breakouts and their severity.

Sometimes when you wake up in the morning, hundreds of whiteheads (which are Demodex worms, which cause baldness), will be standing on end on your face. They are easy to miss, but if you ever look in the mirror and see them standing there, take a dry cotton cloth and gently wipe them away.

Please remember that in the beginning you apply Retin-A over a light layer of moisturizer. This is necessary until your skin acclimates. Wait at least three months from the time you start using Retin-A before you apply it directly to your skin.

When you start to use it directly on your skin, monitor closely, for you may need to use the cream only one or two times a week or even less. Or your skin may be so sensitive you may need to use it only every two weeks at first. Some people have been able to use it everyday from the beginning, and loved their results. Let your skin be the judge.

- When you start using Retin-A directly on your skin, wait five minutes after washing, rub in the Retin-A and apply a thin layer of SRC or your favorite moisturizer immediately. Rubbing Retin-A in produces more intense exfoliating, and thus, quicker results, however, monitor your skin and see which way of using it is best for you.

- Do not place a glob of Retin-A on your skin and leave it there. Do not place a glob of Retin-A on your skin and rub it in.

- Apply Retin-A only at night. If you know you are going to be in the sun for an extended period the next day, do not use Retin-A the night before.

- Make it a point to wash or cleanse your face three times a day for at least 30 days after the last time you use Retin-A. If you remember nothing else, this is the most important thing you need to keep in mind about using Retin-A. Using a moisturizer after washing is pretty important also.

People have all kinds of excuses for not doing this, but it can be easily worked into your routine. Just don't get uptight about it, and do it. Many people say, "I have to work, and I wear makeup; I feel naked without it and I can't wash my face at lunch time because it takes a half an hour to reapply makeup." Well, who says you <u>have</u> to wash your face at lunchtime?

Even glamorous career women who take tons of time applying makeup in the mornings before work can wash their faces three times a day if they cleanse in the morning with their regular shower, in the evening when they come home from work and at night before going to bed. After a year and you are only using exfoliants once a week, or every two or three weeks, washing your face twice a day is sufficient.

Some days I wash my face four or five times a day. This just accelerates the peeling-off process. Let your face tell you how often you can wash or cleanse it. If you have time and can do it five or six times a day, great. Just make sure you are not forcibly peeling the skin off. Allow it to come off gradually with each washing.

When I was working in an office environment I would just duck into the ladies room and wash my face with the soap there, dab on a little blush and SRC and baby powder, and I was set. It took about two minutes. I carry a clean terry cloth in my purse so I can clean my face while away from home, but even in a public bathroom it is relatively easy to wash your face with your hands.

Remember that if you use Retin-A and do not wash your face at least three times a day, your old skin which will be peeling away can become impacted, so make sure you remember to wash at least three times a day. If your life is going to be too hectic to wash three times a day, don't use Retin-A at that time.

Set up a routine for face washing that will be easy to fall into. Morning with the shower, evenings after work and at night before bed. Don't make it complicated.

Many people have reported to me that they like using just the Herbal Lotion all over once a month followed by the Rose Cream daily after a bath or shower and that it did all of the exfoliating and skin repair that they needed because it killed all the parasites that were causing skin problems and malformations in the first place. I have also found this to be true. So you can choose to just use Rose Beauty Cream by rubbing tiny amounts into your face and you will still get a fabulous result: beautiful dewey clear healthy looking skin. For best result to detoxify the body, **The Package** listed on my website will give you 4 products that last one person 3 months to do a basic detox, 21 pages of information on how to detox your home, body, bed and raw foods, how to protect yourself from re-infection, how to clean a hotel bed or guest bed so you don't come away with unwanted critters, what everyone is deficient in, and lost of vital information that you need to start a basic parasite detox. The website is barbarafrank222.com, click on Donate For Products and follow prompts.

Chapter 4

RECOMMENDED
DOSAGE OF RETIN-A

Apply the smallest amount of Retin-A possible to a clean face, one or two minutes after you have applied the tiniest bit of moisturizer. Use enough to cover the width of a pencil eraser head by dotting it on your forehead, cheeks and chin and rubbing it in. If your skin is not especially fragile, you can massage it in for about one minute after you have been using it for a month. If you have terrible acne, discolored skin, wrinkles, freckles, pockmarks and such, rub it in longer. After your skin becomes accustomed to Retin-A (after three months), occasionally massage it in for two or three minutes.

If your skin is oily or olive, you definately need to use my Southern Rose Cream to prevent overpigmentation and keloiding, a condition where the skin over-heals and darkens.

Just remember not to scrub your skin. Scrubbing can cause discoloration. If your skin is allowed to slough off naturally as it will, discoloration does not normally occur. *Cleanse your face three times a day to allow the exfoliating skin to slough off. Always use a moisturizer after washing. Moisturize twice.*

If you take it upon yourself not to use a moisturizer, the results will be unpleasant. Just trust me, try using exfoliants the way I recommend, and you will love it. No one will know you are exfoliating and within a short time, you will see beautiful results.

Very Important
To Remember

Retin-A nor any or the other exfoliants should never be used around the lips, nose and the outward tips of the eyes. Even if you use Retin-A anywhere on your face, it can cause the lips and their edges to peel from the mere action of washing your face because this spreads the exfoliant. As Retin-A is spread all over your face when you wash, and as it is a powerful exfoliant, and the eye tissue is most delicate, it only makes sense that this tissue may begin to peel, and probably more at times. Use SRC and vitamin E oil straight from the capsules to help it heal faster.

If your lips and eyes peel too much, stop using exfoliant for awhile. Remember, too severe peeling means you are going too fast, so slow down with your frequency of use.

Some people have called me terrified because they felt this precious eye skin should not ever be tampered with. However if you check this eye tissue out closely using a mirror and the sun, you will see that it is probably more damaged than any skin on your face because it is so delicate. But what frightened my clients was that they had been brainwashed to believe that this skin can not be handled roughly, and Retin-A was being rough on it.

How else can we get rid of wrinkles? We exfoliate them. Gently. This process will just strengthen those tissues in the long run. To clarify: no exfoliant is to be used in the eye area. After seeing my eye area peel countless times, and seeing the beautiful results, I just let it happen when it happens.

If you have some cortisone cream, a prescription strength is better, then try a little (and I mean use a minuscule amount) of that on the eye area along with the vitamin E oil and SRC. Never slather anything on your face. Use the products I am recommending very frugally.

Do not allow any of the products you use to get into your eyes. Any time you use any cream around your eye area, pat it with baby powder and dust off excess to prevent anything from getting into your eyes. Notice how baby powder keeps eye makeup in place.

If you have a prescription strength of cortisone cream it brings almost immediate relief of dry, painful skin with just a dab. It is especially effective for superficial hemorrhoids or any broken skin, often healing within hours. Do not use frequently.

If you are adamant and do not want your eye area to peel (and after a few times, or even once, some people have felt this way), then wash the eye area first, and separately, from the rest of your face. Use your hands or a clean wash cloth, because the one you washed with yesterday will have traces of exfoliant in it. This way you will not be spreading minute amounts of Retin-A or exfoliant into your eye area.

At any rate, any peeling around the eye, lip and nose area resolves itself rather quickly if the above instructions are followed. If the peeling causes the area around the lips or tips of the eyes to darken, use one of the commercially prepared skin lighteners and apply it lightly to the dark areas only.

> *Monitor Your Skin Closely*
> *At This Stage*

If your skin starts to darken in places, particularly in the places where new skin is appearing, then start using my Southern Rose Cream which will even out the skin tone. This means two things: 1. That you are either scrubbing too hard and peeling off the new skin before it is time, or 2. That you probably need to cleanse more frequently and gentler. In 99% of cases, peeling skin is mites coming out of the blood which Retin A, AHA's and my Rose Cream kill.   In any case, if you know you have a tendency to darken when bruised, you should use SRC as a protective measure since using exfoliant anywhere on the face can cause the skin all over the face to peel. I have experienced poison ivy scars from when I was six years old disappearing from SRC, and others have told me the same. It also minimizes surgical scars.

> *What Are The Alternatives?*

Consider this- if you had surgery to lift your face, which involves having a surgeon pull the skin taut and cut away the excess, besides the pain and healing, you are also out of 3-5,000 dollars, depending on which plastic surgeon you use, because insurance does not cover the procedure. You have to deal with the pain and suffering of having surgery, waiting around in a doctor's office, and you have to take off from work to heal. That is why I say you can be happy to pay 30 dollars for a tube of cream that is going to last a year or two and make you beautiful in the privacy of your own home. And, unlike plastic surgery, the results you get are irreversible!

I have never seen a freckle that did not turn out to be a parasite. Usually, there are hundreds under one freckle, which goes away completely when the parasites are killed.

Chapter 5

> # YOU CAN
> # REVERSE THE
> # RAVAGES OF AGE!

Can you imagine looking younger as you grow older? As I approach fifty, I am often told I look closer to twenty and people become astounded, totally flabbergasted to learn that I have two grandchildren! Yet that is what you will be facing when you join this program, looking younger as you grow older. A doctor examined me and exclaimed that I had the body and urine of a 20-year old!

There is no denying it, looking young has a tremendous effect on the mind and a person's life. If I looked twenty years older than I do now, I would not be doing what I am doing right now in my life, nor having so much fun! Let's face it, this is a youth-oriented society and it is a lot easier to go with the flow than against it.

I discovered by accident thirteen years ago that Retin-A not only got rid of my acne and the unsightly craters created in my face by acne scars, it also got rid of my wrinkles, even my freckles! It helped get rid of the baby fat that caused my face to look puffy, and thus, older. I even discovered I could greatly reduce my cellulite by using it! To test it, I applied it to one half of a scar and that half disappeared! Deep wrinkles take longer to remove, but they will go.

With a lot of creativity, I discovered it **could make me beautiful!**

I stumbled upon a miracle, and learned a mind boggling secret- - that during this time of incredible change, and while my skin was restructuring itself, I could also re-form my face. At first I thought, these changes are not going to stay. But, unbelievably, they did!

As I waited day after day for the effect of what I was doing to go away, it didn't! And with a new sense of awareness I realized it was not going to go away, and also that it was not only not going away, but becoming more pronounced as time passed.

I watched myself becoming more and more beautiful, and it was as if a miracle were occurring. It was, and I was making it happen. This incredible information has changed my life and can change yours too!

> ### What To Do With The.
> ### Uglies

Give your ugliness to Retin-A or one of the other exfoliants. I got rid of all my ugly skin with it. Use Retin-A on your neck, under your chin, on fat legs and thighs, and you won't believe how tight they become after a week and how silky they become after a month! If there is a particularly sagging or ugly spot that you want to remove, rub Retin-A in longer there.

All in all, your use of Retin-A should be very, very small. Do not rub large amounts of tretonin into your skin under any condition. This will not speed up the exfoliating process and could result in damage to your skin.

Some of the things that Retin-A nor any other exfoliant will not work on are mites or parasites. Make sure you are not suffering from any such condition. I will mention two: scabies, which comes from a mite (*Sarcopets scabiei*) and Rosacea which has been around for years (remember W. C. Fields?) and which scientists just discovered comes from a mite.

Both are disturbingly common and highly infectious, so don't blame yourself if you have picked up one of these parasites. They can literally ruin your skin. The National Geographic has made a video about them, called The Body Snatchers. The following is from their website entitled The Body Snatchers. "...Existing as a parasite is the most common way of life on Earth. Every creature has parasites- parasites even live on other parasites. In short, we cannot escape or ignore the effects and dangers of these tiny life-forms. In fact, parasites have killed more humans than all the wars in history.[3] The website is http://www.nationalgeographic.com/tv/explorer/exp012200.html. Scabies, one of the most common, is characterized by skin eruptions and itching, Rosacea by redness and eruptions of the skin. I have developed the only all natural treatment for eliminating them that I know of, and have treated thousands for them in my clinic. Breast tumors are caused by mites and I have had success eliminating them by simply eliminating mites. All the people who came to me with breast tumors reported that mites came out and the tumors got smaller and smaller as they massaged the mites away. A list of people is available upon request. Just write me in care of the publisher.

If you choose to use an abrasive, use a skin lightener the first few times just to make sure your skin does not discolor. This is especially true for dark-skinned individuals, who almost always over-heal or keloid, and especially for Blacks and yellow-skinned individuals who have a tendency to keloid.

> *You Can Have Ice Cream*
> *With Cherries And Whipped*
> *Cream On Top! Even*
> *Sprinkles!*

I use this metaphor to demonstrate that you can have it all! Don't hold back! Think of your transformation as something that you get the opportunity to do to make yourself absolutely gorgeous. And since the small amount of work you are going to perform to be beautiful is not going to take very much of your time, think of the minutes you spend peeling away your ugly old skin as precious moments that you are lucky enough to get to have because of what it is going to give you. For is it not true that if you were not peeling it off, the ugly or undesirable skin would still be there?

After all, you could have spent the rest of your life not knowing about how to look younger and more beautiful and just aged naturally along with the rest of the uninformed population.

---

[3]   Copyright Explorer TV@ National Geographic.com January 22, 2000.

Moisturizers For The Hair

Shiny, bouncy hair can make anyone appear more attractive. Keep a shower cap or quart-sized bag in your shower. Once a week after you put conditioner on, pile your hair on top of your head and tuck under the shower cap or bag and as you shower let the warm water run over the top of your head. To warm your hair quicker, rub your hands along the outside after you first put your hair under to get the warmth in and keep it in longer for extra conditioning. This few minutes of heat causes your conditioner to penetrate deeply. You won't believe the body and silkiness of your hair!

Once or twice a month, immediately after washing your hair, apply a quarter sized drop of conditioner, the ones that contain silicone work best. Part I of my Southern Rose Cream will grow hair and cause the hair to be thicker and fuller than ever. Within ten days hair will appear on bald spots. Continued use will restore the hair unless the baldness was caused by a cut or burn.

Rub the one you choose in your hands before applying it by rubbing it as evenly as you can into your hair. Apply it before any setting lotion or styling gel to lock moisture and shine in. Only a small amount is needed. If your hair turns out too flat, you used too much. If you use a small dab, your hair will be thicker and bouncier! You will love it!

To prevent breakage of your hair, comb it out after you put the conditioner on starting at the ends and work your way up.

Some of the new conditioners contain silicone, a natural ingredient that is very beneficial to the hair. Silicone comes from the mineral silica, which has been used in hair products for years because it helps hair repair itself by smoothing the cuticle. The new products contain more silicone than the old ones and work 100 times better!

Smoothing the hair cuticle enables light to bounce off the hair. Silicone also repels moisture and combats the frizzies. You can get pure silicone from the pharmacy inexpensively. Apply it in very small amounts same as recommended for the Alberto VO5 conditioning hairdressing. Remember, applying too much makes the hair look flat.

I actually got better results using some of the commercially prepared silicone-containing products such as John Frieda's Frizz-Ease. Some others are Altobella's Maximum Shine Gel, Alberto Frizz Solver and Shine Enhancer, L'Oreal's Colorvive Technicare Daily Color Sealer, Sebastian Systema Laminates Spray, Aveda Purefume Brilliant Spray On For Hair, Dep's Shine Conditioner and Jheri Redding's Polisher and his Extra Reflections Polisher Mousse. Aura's Leave-On Conditioning Elixir is especially good for Black hair.

Many of the new silicone-containing products do not say they contain silicone. If you see "one" in the end of a word in the ingredients, that usually means silicone, and gloss, shine or glass in the name is a good indication that a product contains silicone.

Chapter 6

HOW TO RE-SHAPE YOUR FACE TO BE MORE ATTRACTIVE

Water is the most hydrating substance on earth. It is known for its ability to change the surface of rocks. Clean water on the skin moisturizes, heals and nourishes it.

Every time you wash your face you super-hydrate your skin. Imagine what increasing washing from once to three times a day will do to improve the appearance of your skin! Now you are going to learn how to use water to re-moisturize and re-shape your face.

I discovered that if I held water firmly against my skin and re-formed my face the way I wished it looked, my appearance started to change. I pushed in on the concave area under my cheeks to heighten my cheekbones. I gently pulled and re-formed my eyes and they have actually grown and become more oblong, and the effect is doe-like, and beautiful.

You will get best results if you hold your face in water for at least three minutes everyday. This is one of the special things I do for myself because I have seen the difference when I do it and when I don't.

The best time to re-form your face is at night before going to bed. After you wash your face, cup your hand with water and hold it to your face to re-form areas that you want to re-shape, like your cheekbones and eyes.

Hold the position until all the water runs out of your hand. Repeat one to three times. Even doing this for one minute a day will make a big difference in the appearance and texture of your skin!

A simple way to re-form your face is to stand so that the shower water splashes onto your face while employing the acupressure technique for *Facial Beauty* in Chapter 3 using all your fingers. For the sake of water conservation, do not do this for more than one minute.

This is the time to raise your cheekbones, pull back your eyes and soften wrinkles. Slowly and gently pull back on your eyes, then gently raise your cheekbones by pressing gently under each cheekbone, holding the water tightly yet gently to your face and actually shaping your face the way you would like it to look. Everything you do to your face to re-form it should be painless.

I also like the results I get from re-forming my face using a natural sponge soaked with water. I bury my face in it while emphasizing my cheeks and eyes and leave it there until the sponge needs to be soaked again.

Except for when I take a shower or do a facial, I almost always wash my face with cold tap water. The cold stimulates circulation and tightens pores. It is ideal for re-molding the skin, although warm water can work well also. Using warm water first for re-forming your face and cold water in the end is very effective for re-shaping the face. Cold water seems to make the exfoliation process go smoother also.

During and after washing is the best time to change and re-mold your face. I made myself have high cheekbones and beautiful huge almond shaped eyes by simply re-molding my face and eyes with lukewarm and cold water, a cotton cloth and my hands.

The shape of your eyes is moldable and you can change how they look. Even though you are fully grown, your eyes still are sensitive to growth factors, which means the shape of them can be changed. Growth factors are the chemicals that stimulate growth.

According to an article in The New York Times entitled **Big Eyes**, under which there is a question:

Do your eyes grow? the answer to the question is:
"Dr. Hendrickson pointed out that the eye is still moldable and can change its shape."[8]

If you never heard of this, I have developed a technique that you can use to change the shape of your eyes. Listen to how it is done: During and after

---

[8] © 1992 by The New York Times Company. Reprinted by permission.

thoroughly cleansing your face and neck by washing briskly (depending on if your skin can take being washed briskly), soak a cloth (folded in three or four layers), and hold it to your face and gently but firmly mold your cheeks and eyes the way you would like them to look. You will notice a small change in your appearance even the first time you do this. Tilt your head back if possible, so you are working with gravity.

Press your cheeks in as you wash and rinse. If you have time do not dry your face. It is helpful to press in on the indentations under your cheeks for a full 30 seconds after washing. After you have re-formed your face for about one minute, let the water evaporate for maximum hydration. Try this process with a wash cloth and without, using just your hands.

Push in on the concave area under your cheeks to heighten your cheekbones. There should never be any pain while doing any of these processes. Gently pull and re-form the skin at the far corners of your eyes and your eyes actually will become more elongated, giving you that doe-like innocent look of wide-eyed beauty.

Gently pull the corners of your eyes back during and after washing your face. Hold for ten seconds at a time. After you have done this for about two months, you will notice that your face has taken on a new form. This is a gradual process that pays off!

I have become convinced that exfoliating brings growth factors to the face, and thus, allows this transformation to be possible.

Once you have established the look you want, you don't have to keep re-forming your face every time you wash it. Once a day after your shower should be sufficient. Sometimes I do it once a week since my look is set. It took approximately two months of re-forming my face to change my looks.

Look at yourself in the mirror and analyze what would be needed to make you more attractive. Almost anyone will benefit from widened eyes, thinner noses and higher cheekbones.

The next time you wash your face, gently, ever so gently, pull your eyes back and you will elongate them. Gently press your fingers in directly on the indentations under your cheekbones. Make sure there is no pain or discomfort. Remember, gently is the only way to do this re-forming process. You're going to love how this process will change your looks.

Yes, noses can be pinched, and darker makeup can be applied to the sides of your nose to make it look slimmer. Other cases require a plastic surgeon. Even the worst noses can benefit from crimping with the fingers during the shower. However, 95 percent of your time spent re-forming your face should be spent on re-forming your cheekbones and eyes.

I do this by pressing my four fingers under my cheekbones and pushing the skin under my cheeks in and heightening my cheeks. I use all four of my fingers, fanning them around to my ears, and I gently hold them there. This has made a tremendous difference in further emphasizing my cheekbones. Please remember to take a picture of yourself at the beginning of this therapy so you can gage in a year how much it has changed your appearance. Questions on this technique are welcome! Just write to me in care of the publisher.

I had a slight double chin which I got rid of completely by using Retin-A. If you have this problem, try using Retin-A on the lower part of your face and neck and notice the difference after a month.

Here is a photograph of me before I started my metamorphosis:

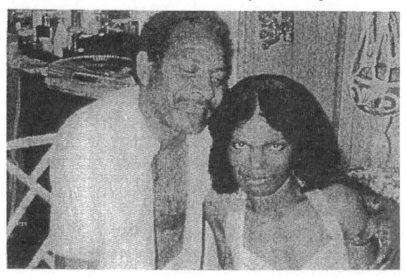

As you can see by my cover photograph, these techniques have changed my appearance and thus, my life!

I started experimenting with Retin-A and studying its use, and it even grows hair! It stimulates the skin to rejuvenate itself by peeling off the old skin and stimulating the skin to make new cells, even, miraculously, new collagen, leaving behind brand new beautiful baby skin composed of young, plump cells. New blood vessels form and the increased flow of blood, along with the new tighter cells, gives your skin a rosy glow. Exfoliants are *one of the most incredible discoveries of this century!*

It certainly makes one think that if such a substance can stimulate the cells to renew themselves, then it may be possible to rejuvenate all of the body's cells. Actually, contrary to what has been long held to be true, that rejuvenation is not often possible in humans, new research is finding that in a lot of cases, it is possible.

A human liver will grow back if a part of it is cut away. This proves that our bodies have the capability to regenerate. Thinking things can't happen often prevents them from happening.

Researchers find that people who believe they can recover, even when doctors say there is no way, strangely recover. The most important single factor that contributes to remarkable recoveries is the person's state of mind.

Beliefs Held To Be Key To Longevity[9]

Studies show that people in nursing homes keep themselves alive until after their anniversary, Christmas or their granddaughter's birthday. More than 6,000 people claim to have been cured miraculously after visiting the healing waters at Lourdes, France.

Yet researchers find that the most incredible thing about them is their belief in God and/or the cure. The only unusual thing about the water is that it has large amounts of naturally-occurring hydrogen peroxide.

In fact, a whole new science, Psychoneuroimmunology, the role of mind, feelings and beliefs on health and healing has evolved.

---

[9] © 1993 by The New York Times Company. Reprinted by permission.

An article in **The Washington Post** proclaims:

Experiments Suggest Brain Cells Regenerate

Finding In Mice Challenges Long-Held Belief.
"Cell biologists have found evidence that challenges one of the most widely accepted beliefs in biology."[10]

Hearing-Loss Study Hints At Reviving Cells

"Scientists have shown that sensory hair cells in the inner ear of mammals, which are important in hearing and balance, can regenerate after being damaged. It has long been thought that the loss was irreversible in humans and other mammals."[11]

Reading the articles from experts who felt Retin-A was wonderful as I did had a tremendous impact on me (although by the time I read them, I already knew the power of Retin-A), because now I had a vehicle to convince my sisters of its power! A respected authority was saying the same thing that I had been telling them for years!

I sent copies of articles about Retin-A to all three of my sisters. They could not understand how I was able to look so young, yet they did not take me seriously when I told them how I did it. After reading the articles, they all immediately got tubes of Retin-A, even sent me one. Next time I saw them (a year later) I was amazed at the improvements.

My younger sister who has dry skin got a prescription and refilled it until she had a tube for all three of her sisters. Her wrinkles were worse than any of ours, although I had the worst acne. When I saw her again the heavy lines around her mouth were almost gone, and she had a smug smile like someone who had

---

[10]   © 1992 by The Washington Post, Washington, DC. Reprinted with permission. By Boyce Rensberger.

[11]   © 1993 by The New York Times Company. Reprinted by permission.

cheated on time. My older sister who had grown to look perpetually tired from the sagging facial skin around her mouth looked remarkably firmer and fresher.

Chapter 7

HOW TO CHANGE THE CONTOURS OF YOUR FACE

If you want to make the skin between the end of your nose and your ear lobe more taut try this: use one finger to rub Retin-A in a straight line from the end of your nose to the end of your ear lobe on clean, moisturized skin. This will cause only the skin in that area to peel off, thus it will grow taut and you will begin to see the contour of your cheekbone even if you have never seen it before.

Just to clarify, rub the Retin-A in a straight line from the end of your nose to your ear lobe every night for one week. Rub it in for two or three minutes for maximum effect. Rub very slowly, gently, but firmly. Within a week, if you wash and re-form your face three times a day (with morning shower, evening after work and at night before bed, and you can get the routine down to two minutes), you will see a dramatic difference.

Continue for two or three weeks and the effect will be even more noticeable. Use the acupressure points *Facial Beauty* nightly to further the effect of your contour.

If you decided you cannot use Retin-A, an alpha-hydroxy acid-containing moisturizer can be used in place of it. Make sure to keep away from around eyes, nose and mouth.

Think of the delicious possibilities. How would you like to re-form your face to look? If you are having any doubts about this technique, let me assure you that it does work and anyone, no matter how attractive or unattractive, can make theirself more attractive using it.

The most effective time to re-form your face is during and after washing. Look in the mirror and gently pull the outer ends of your eyes back. You look more exotic. Gently press three inches under your eyes on your cheekbones and ever so gently push your cheeks back.

After you have decided what changes you would like to make, re-form your face at least once a day. You need only one minute of re-forming your face a day to make an incredible difference in how you look. When you shower, wet your face first for maximum hydration and keep it wet during the entire process. This will help the tightening and peeling-off process also.

- Wash your face with a cotton terry cloth. Gently pull back on your eyes. The water does not have to be on your face, but warm water followed by starkly cold water is most effective in the re-molding process. You can do this in or out of the shower.

- For the sake of water conservation, please do most of your re-forming and re-shaping after the shower, preferably with a clean sink full of cold water. It also helps to work with gravity. Make sure not to press too hard on your face to prevent any nerve damage. Make sure your re-forming of your face is painless.

- Alternate using the washcloth and your hands to re-form your face. Or try using just your hands for one week, or just the washcloth to see which method is more effective. You may decide you prefer one over the other or both methods to re-form your face.

The change will happen faster if you can re-form your face every time you wash it. Even if you only have thirty seconds to spend re-forming your face, that thirty seconds once or twice a day will cause an incredible change after one month!

Work washing your face three times a day into your routine and forget about it. Cleansing your face with Cetaphil three times a day is a good way to get your three exfoliations in per day. You can massage the Cetaphil in for two or three minutes if you have time, re-forming as you massage. When you use Cetaphil, you can see the old skin come off, for it wipes away.

Using Cetaphil presents an excellent opportunity to re-form and exfoliate at the same time. Since Cetaphil speeds the process, the peeling of the old skin will accelerate.

When you apply Retin-A you can apply it in ways that will accentuate your facial features. Long, slow, horizontal strokes work best.

To help get rid of a sagging neck, apply to your chin and under your chin for one week or two. Keep away from lips.

Another way to lift your face is by applying Retin-A up the sides of your face to the temples. Remember the contours you want to create in your face as you wash it. This gives you the power to replicate success. Use the water you wash your face with to help you mold it to be more beautiful.

Facial Beauty 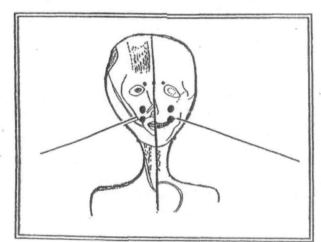 *Facial Beauty*

Chapter 8

HOW TO GET AN
INSTANT FACE
LIFT

Two minutes after applying moisturizer to a clean face rub Retin-A around the circumference of your face about one to one-half inches in diameter around the hairline. Massage in for two minutes. For best results do this in early evening around 8 p.m. or the last time you wash your face before going to bed.

Repeat the application of Retin-A around the outer edge of your face for five to seven days, making sure to rub in for at least two minutes for maximum effect. Within a week, if you wash your face three times a day (with morning shower, evening after work and at night before bed), you will see a dramatic difference.

You can get the routine of washing your face, applying blush and moisturizer down to two or three minutes.

While washing your face, mold it the way you want it, either using your finger tips or the cotton cloth. Neutrogena is a superior soap for this peeling-off process. Rose soaps seems to moisturize and refine pores. Sea Breeze is excellent for over-porosity.

Revlon Honey Masque mixed with an equal amount of their Whole-Egg Masque is a superior masque and pore refiner. Blend the two in the palm of your hand. Apply, keeping away from eyes. For best results, leave on for about thirty minutes or until dry. Follow with nothing, for the masque moisturizes. If you must use foundation, it shortens the life of what the masque accomplishes.

If you want to raise your cheeks overnight, simply rub Retin-A under your cheeks and rub from cheek to ear. Also apply Retin-A from the ear to the middle of the forehead on both sides. Next morning when you wash your face, re-form it by gently but firmly pushing in three inches under your eyes on your cheekbones. There should be no discomfort. Use warm water to wash, then cold water for re-forming.

A sleep mask is also good for occasional use.

For Quicker Results

If you want your skin to be more taut, leave your face wet during your entire shower and notice how much tighter your skin feels. Washing your face three times a day is mandatory in order to get the maximum benefit from using exfoliants. The peeling will commence smoothly if you simply take a few minutes and wash your face those three times.

The acupressure points for *Facial Beauty* also help re-form the cheekbones.

Chapter 9

> # HOW TO USE RETIN-A
> # TO MAKE YOUR BACK,
> # THIGHS AND
> # BUTTOCKS BEAUTIFUL

Use Retin-A or the exfoliant of your choice on these areas the same as you use it on your face. Do not worry about washing your back, thighs and buttocks three times a day. Since they are not as noticeable or accessible it is okay to wash them once a day. There was a drastic reduction in the visibility of the cellulite that had been on the back of my thighs for years after I used Retin-A on it. I found that the more I rubbed it in, the more it seemed to get rid of the cellulite.

That is because Retin-A causes the outer layer of skin to fall off and makes the under layer (dermis, which contains collagen that gives skin its elasticity and youthfulness) make more of everything. What you end up with is a new beginning, a beautiful newly regenerated skin!

Because the skin on your thighs is different from that on your face, a stronger strength of Retin-A or AHA can be used in most cases. Do the patch test on your thighs before starting treatment. Use Retin-A very frugally, same as on your face. If you have two strengths, use one on each thigh for the patch test.

I had been running for more than twenty-five years and still the cellulite remained in my thighs. Now my thighs look like twenty-five year old thighs. I do not know if the effect would be so dramatic in a person fifty or one hundred pounds overweight. I was only about fifteen pounds overweight, so tightening this skin was not difficult at all. On my thighs and buttocks I use the stronger strength of Retin-A, the one with the red label, 0.01 percent. I massage it in for three or four minutes.

Use Retin-A on these areas no more than a week at a time, then allow a peeling-off period. I allow two or three weeks, then use it for several days, or another week depending on how my skin reacts.

If you use a loofa or buf puf on your thighs and buttocks, use with extreme caution until your skin becomes accustomed to it. Unlike the face, a loofa or buf puf it can be used on a pimply back that you are using exfoliant on. Gentle is the word. Glide it over your skin, especially your buttocks, to remove butt bumps. This in conjunction with exercise and massage will firm and tone your thighs so that they are gorgeous. And your buttocks and thighs will feel like silk.

Massage is excellent for toning and firming the thighs also. Swimming, running, dancing, stretching and Yoga-type exercises will speed the toning process.

You can get the same result cheaper by simply applying the Natural Herbal Lotion to the areas where you want to get rid of cellulite and varicose veins. You will find that these conditions are caused by parasites as well. Just put undiluted Natural Herbal Lotion on the affected areas once a week and follow by rubbing undiluted Rose Beauty Cream all over the areas after a bath or shower. You will find tiny microbes coming out of the areas and after a time, depending on how long the condition has been there, you will see the skin becoming clear and the cellulite going away. For varicose veins you just rub the critters out most effectively after a bath or shower when the pores are open. Sometimes the parasites will overgrow in the veins so much they make it explode. But as long as they keep coming out, you should just keep rubbing them for a few minutes a day.

Chapter 10

HOW TO GET RID
OF DARK CIRCLES
UNDER THE EYES

While still in my teens I noticed the ugly dark circles under my eyes that caused me to look raccoonish and weird. Greatly alarmed by this for I had emerged from ugly duckling to normal looking, and looking normal after being called the ugly duckling was very important to me.

I became a detective, investigating and trying to solve this mysterious dire situation. I could not believe that glaring dark circles had managed to creep up without my knowledge and grow under both my eyes. I had to find a solution, and quick! *Dark circles under the eyes can be an indication of a serious health (liver) condition. Make sure you are not suffering from such a condition.*

Further investigation revealed that the eyeliner I used and failed to wash off at night was seeping into my skin and causing the discoloration. I resolved to remove my eye makeup every night.

At the library I found out that tea bags soaked and placed under the eyes did wonders for dark circles.

Since diet has everything to do with appearance, especially the appearance of the skin, I enhanced my diet to mostly fruits, vegetables, legumes and plenty of fluids, all of which help eliminate dark circles under the eyes.

Allium cepa, the onion, when used as a homeopathic preparation, cures watery eyes that cause dark circles under the eyes because the eyes are being rubbed. Check with your homeopathic pharmacist with your exact symptoms for the correct dosage. Or check in your homeopathic pharmacy's Materia Medica for the proper remedy according to your symptoms.

Hay fever can cause rubbing of the eyes, which can cause dark circles. Hay fever is usually an indication of an underlying chronic weakness, and therefore it is recommended that you see a homeopathic doctor. Try a homeopathic dose of mixed pollen for relief.

Some women are really beautiful, but dark circles under their eyes spoil it all and give them a sort of living-dead look. Sometimes dark circles can be caused by too much protein. Try a low-protein, high carbohydrate diet. Of course that means plenty of vegetables and fruits also.

Vitamin and mineral deficiencies can cause dark circles under the eyes. Make sure you get a good, balanced vitamin and mineral supplement. Take evening primrose oil and watch your dark circles disappear.

Two other things that worked to get rid of my dark circles was using sunless tanning lotion and skin lightener simultaneously. Here's how:

Apply a small film of skin lightener to the dark circle. Be careful not to apply too close to the eye. A Q-Tip is perfect for this, Right under that, where the dark circle ends, apply the sunless tanning lotion. Allow to dry. Make sure to pat with powder. After a week, or sooner, you will see beautiful results.

This last solution should be used temporarily, for it's too much trouble to do everyday. How long should you use this last process? As long as it works for you and you are careful about keeping chemicals out of your eyes.

Chapter 11

WHAT MAKES THOSE UGLY WRINKLES ANYWAY?

To know what causes them is the key to getting rid of them. Actually if you look closely at a wrinkle in a mirror with the sun on your face you will see that the wrinkle is usually composed of hundreds of tiny whiteheads, which are really mites, Demodex.

Most people will want to go right in and squeeze them out since they are nothing but crap. This will be a mistake because they have to be prepared before they are removed. You can not afford to damage the skin around the pimple.

Why sweat it? Another option is just to allow Southern Rose Cream, Retin-A or one of the other exfoliants take care of them. Since you are going to be peeling off the top layer of skin, you can wait until the exfoliant removes them. That is the safest and most logical option. So what if it takes longer? You do not run the risk of damaging your skin.

People who get too much sun as well as people who stay indoors too much can get leathery skin. Vitamin C, vitamin E and vitamin A preserve the natural suppleness and moisture of the skin. Research has shown that vitamin C makes the skin make new collagen, one of the essential ingredients of healthy skin.

When you start taking vitamins and minerals you will notice that your health will improve, you will have more energy, your thinking will become clearer, your eyesight will improve, but unless you have a serious illness, nothing will improve as much as your skin. In fact, one of the most important contributors to good skin is nutrition. For years we have known that vitamins A and zinc contribute greatly to good skin.

Now we know that there are a wide array of nutrients as well as foods that contribute to good skin. If there is not enough vitamin A in the diet, the corners of the mouth begin to peel. Amino acids and copper help preserve the elasticity of the skin.

Wrinkles, and particularly the ones around the eyes, respond well to Chamomile. Use Chamomile lotion from a homeopathic pharmacy to help smooth wrinkles and fine lines around your eyes and on your entire face.

It used to be that the only alternative women had against wrinkles was to pump themselves up with steroids. But there is a female hormone, progesterone, which has a long-term beneficial effect on the skin. It prevents the aging of collagen.

You can get this hormone by eating sesame seeds. Just sprinkle them on your salad everyday. Taking them in this way can also slow or prevent menopause and vaginal dryness. Replacing estrogen is not for people who have health problems or family histories that prevent it or adverse effects from the treatment.

Progesterone is known for stabilizing the autoimmune system. This prevents the drying of skin caused by aging. The body makes progesterone when we eat liver (I recommend eating organic liver only), eggs, and sweet potatoes. Only recently, it was discovered that estrogen, also found in sesame seeds, helps prevent Alzheimers. It is also essential for the developing fetus's brain.

Chapter 12

SOME OTHER
THINGS THAT
CAUSE WRINKLES

One of them is how you sleep. Notice that you sleep most comfortably in a certain position. Does that position have you putting pressure on one side of your face? That sleeping position could be adding unnecessary wrinkles and signs of aging to your face. This can sometimes make your face asymmetrical. Also, your hair grows slower on the side of your head that you sleep on.

To find out if your face has become asymmetrical, cover one side with a sheet of paper and look at each side to see which one looks like it is being slept on. Notice the position you wake up in to see if you are sleeping on your face.

If you are, gradually get yourself out of the habit of sleeping that way. Yes you can do it. You can even sleep in a way that will enhance your looks. If you can sleep face up, gravity pulls your skin in the direction you want it to be in for a youthful appearance.

After sleeping on my stomach for years (in order to have a flat stomach, and by the way, it works, but there are prices to pay like stiff neck and lumps in breasts) I decided after having the benign lump removed from my breast that I really wasn't happy sleeping that way anyway and that I needed a new way to sleep.

I read about sleeping for beauty by sleeping spread eagle so that gravity pulled on the skin in the desired direction. I had to gradually get myself accustomed to doing it, but now I actually love sleeping that way because I know it helps make me beautiful and it feels so free. I hung a picture of the universe over my bed, and in some of my dreams, I'm out there exploring it!

Freud made some reference to people who sleep on their backs as being extremely well adjusted. So there are psychological factors involved in the way you sleep.

● Smoking causes wrinkles. It depletes the body of life-giving oxygen and essential vitamins and minerals, which keep skin looking young.

● Another thing that causes wrinkles is not eating enough life-giving foods like bananas, cucumbers, strawberries, apples, carrots, broccoli, and other fruits and vegetables.

● Laughing too much causes wrinkles. It leaves lines in your face if it is done too often. Some people walk around with a smile on their face. And it stays there.

● The way you wear your face can cause wrinkles. If you get stuck on a frown, if you are always pondering your life's problems, the wrinkle from the frown and pondering will be left on your face. If you keep those little worry lines on your face they will make their home there. Some people frown so much, fighting off the problems and perils of life, that they wear, embedded in their foreheads, the wrinkles from this frowning.

● Everyone knows that sun causes wrinkles, so keep it off of your face for extended periods. More than five minutes of full sun is too much, even if you are using an AHA and sunscreen.

Chapter 13

> # *LEARN SOMETHING*
> # *FROM BABIES*

Many people don't know it but baby powder is an excellent source for soaking up excess oil from the skin. I often wear no foundation at all, but simply use a cosmetic sponge to apply a light coat of baby powder. After about one or two minutes it will soak in, and the excess can be wiped away with a cosmetic brush or clean cloth. It takes away every trace of shine, soaks up about ten times its weight in oil, de-emphasizes freckles and ugly blotches and emphasizes the beautiful contours of your face.

> *Frame Of Mind And The*
> *State We Put Ourselves In*

Have you ever noticed that children, even young babies, are in a constant state of experiencing life with a fresh, unbiased outlook? Every moment for them is a miracle of discovery and bliss. They smile when you look at them, and are generally in a bubbly, happy state for no apparent reason at all. No one has to tell the child to be happy, he just does it. He is spontaneous, guileless, eager to please and usually open to compromise. What changes all that?

Either *consciously or unconsciously,* we are always in one state or another. Children seem to automatically revert to the positive. Adults generally revert to the negative when they allow their brains to go on automatic. I think that is because in life, we get stuck on the negative experiences, failing to realize that most things go right. But children, in their pure, unspoiled state naturally fit the healthy-minded role model: exhibiting a positive state of mind spontaneously, experiencing ecstasy with and a zest for life, having willingness to compromise and a straightforward, unpretentious demeanor.

You can consciously choose to remain optimistic and childlike even in the face of all kinds of adversity. You simply need to shrink the negative and put it out of your mind and focus on what is positive and what you can change and salvage.

Don't allow yourself to get caught up in life's negativity and frenetics. Step back and away from them. Realize that shit happening is a part of life. You know Murphy's Law, things *will* go wrong! As Buddha said, "Life is suffering." Things going wrong do not change the fact that life is a celebration! And there is not enough time in the day anyway, so you don't want to focus energy on things that have already happened that can not be changed and things that you are powerless over.

As soon as you realize that you can focus your mind on accomplishing goals you want to accomplish instead of just letting it run wild, guess what? That's what will happen with just a little effort from you! Your mind will no longer run wild because you will be directing your energies where you want them.

And as you focus on the things you want and weave plans for attaining them do not stray too far from this truth: Life is a gift and a blessing. Since everything in life happens to teach us an important lesson, rejoice in adversity as a chance for growth and change.

When you think of the fact that any of us could have ended up in another dimension, as, for example, one of the discharged sperm that did not make it to the egg, or an aborted fetus, you can see that every person on earth has a lot to be thankful for, and we should never lose sight of this perspective.

Savor the fact that you don't have cancer, or AIDS, or are not waiting for an organ transplant. We need to be as open and honest as children and stop playing games with one another. Human relationships are the treasure of life. Children and babies know this without ever being told.

PART 2

HOW TO ADD 10 YEARS TO YOUR LIFE NATURALLY

Health is a precious thing...the only thing indeed that deserves to be pursued at the expense not only of time, sweat, labor, worldly goods, but of life itself; since without health life becomes a burden and an affliction.

-MONTAIGNE

Chapter 14

FIRST THINGS FIRST

We have known for many years now that cleanliness can make the difference between health and illness. All you have to do is study history and see the devastation to humans from germs (strep, ecoli), parasites (malaria, encephalitis,) viruses[12] (AIDS, herpes[13]), bacteria (cholera, toxic shock syndrome) and environmental toxins (petrochemicals[14], bleach, ammonia) to realize the validity of this statement.

Years after the devastations to humanity from illnesses and diseases, we discovered that a lot of scourges and illness could have been averted if people had done a simple thing like wash their hands between patients or operations, or boil the milk to kill parasites, or cook the meat fully before eating it.

For a long time mankind did not know that washing hands after going to the bathroom could prevent illness. Knowing how germs and disease are spread has made it important for me to keep my hands clean.

No, I don't think of this world as a hazardous place filled with germs that are going to get me. I think it is a wonderful place where we can live in peace, harmony and bliss if we followed the laws of nature and natural living. Trust me,

---

[12]   Viruses used to be classified as extremely small and therefore airborne, and very contagious, but, apparently, the Centers For Disease Control are still saying that AIDS, which comes from a virus, is not airborne.

[13]   Herpes I is a form of chicken pox that occurs as a fever blister around the rim of the lip, although it can erupt on the actual lip as well. Every fever blister is herpes, whether brought on by sun or food. Herpes II is the genital variety which you can get from having oral sex with someone with herpes I. Both are transmissible for six weeks before and after they erupt and are highly itchy and contagious.

[14]   An overload of petrochemicals in the body could be toxic, producing nausea, fatigue, insomnia, blurred vision, strange aches and pains and depression. Petrochemical byproducts are stored in our fatty tissues until they can be detoxified and excreted by our liver.

heaven does exist on earth and one of the doors to it is enlightenment. Some others are scents and sensory perceptions.

Exercise, proper nutrition, focusing on our commitment to ourselves and our lives can channel a wayward life into a life of prosperity. Enlightenment has transformed me. Heightening my awareness and studying philosophy set off a charge in me. What turns you on? Not many other things can compare to it for bringing you joy. (See Chapter 27 on Awareness.)

Yet disease can pop up and put an end to anyone's joy. Being beautiful means nothing if your health is bad.

Following is a brief description of what we have learned down through the ages about disease and its causes:

We discovered that diseases are generally caused by bacteria or viruses, tiny microscopic organisms that invade the body. Pasteur was one of the first to discover this process. He discovered that people transmitted diseases and viruses among themselves and hygienic practices could help eliminate the spread of many diseases.

We have learned that it will take many years after exposure to a cancer-causing substance for any symptoms of cancer to appear. We have also learned that we can prevent the cancer that someone was exposed to by building up their immune system, eating nourishing anti-oxidative foods and ensuring that their bodies are properly nourished and not just filled up with empty calories.

We now know that exercise is the fountain of youth, that state of mind and beliefs often determine how long a person lives and the quality of their life. We know that repressing emotions and not resolving emotional dilemmas can lead to illness and disease.

You will discover the interventions you can implement to counter disease. After reading countless articles on the importance of keeping the hands clean, especially before eating with them, and especially after handling pets or animals, I realized the importance of good hygiene to my health. I cut my rate for catching colds from two or three a year to one every five or six years.

We have learned why is it so important not to catch colds or introduce toxins and bacteria into our bodies. These conditions weaken our immune systems, make us sick and leave us vulnerable to other infections.

Contrary to what has been popularly believed for decades, according to an article in the Washington Post with the headline:

Washing Hands Can Be A Major Disease-Stopper--As Grandma Knew

"This is because bacteria and viruses, including the strains of virus believed to be responsible for the common cold, are transmitted largely by hand contact from person to person-not by inhalation, as has been believed down through the ages."

"In 20th-century America, the old saying "living from hand to mouth" can be reworked as "dying from hand to mouth" for maybe 80,000 people a year, estimates the federal Centers for Disease Control in Atlanta."

"More than 20,000 deaths a year result directly from infections acquired in a hospital - called nosocomial infections-the CDC reports. These infections contribute indirectly to another 60,000 deaths, the CDC says, and present to the bill-paying public an annual cost of 2.5 billion dollars for treatment, says the Department of Health and Human Services."[15]

Childbed Fever And Hand Washing read the headline in the Washington Post on March 23, 1993. It further stated that:

"It was the unsanitary procedures of doctors that bestowed the deadly gift, its bacteria invading and infecting the reproductive organs, bringing high fever, nausea and severe abdominal pain. . . .and not until the second half of the 20th century would childbed fever enter the rare-disease category in developed countries."[16]

There are even harmful parasites, one of which is Schistosoma mannsoni in the soil and on the ground that can bore through your skin and travel through your bloodstream to live in your guts for the rest of your life. These parasites can go undetected for years and during the course of those years, they impair your health. An article in The New York Times with the headline:

---

[15]   © 1985 by The Washington Post, Washington, DC. Reprinted with permission.

[16]   © 1992 by The Washington Post, Washington, DC. Reprinted with permission.

Worm Uses Hormone Of the Immune System To Infect and Multiply It further states:

"The worms cause schistosomiasis, a parasitic disease that has persisted for centuries and that afflicts an estimated 200 million people. When a person steps into the water the larvae rush over to burrow into their skin.[17]"

These worms use a human hormone to help establish themselves in your body. They bore through the skin and go inside your blood stream and live their entire lives there where they spend all their time living a grand life, as they constantly eat and multiply. Their eggs are sealed in granulomas, which attach to the liver and damage it.

They live off of you and steal essential nutrients that your body needs, and they grow into a tumor-like growth there on your liver. These kinds of parasites can do untold harm to a human fetus. Pets compound these kind of health problems a hundredfold, for they bring along with them their own assortment of parasites and diseases.

Thus, it is advised that if you plan to have children, avoid putting your hands in dirt or going barefoot. The parasites you might pick up could damage your offspring.

Again, the point here is that knowledge is power. As long as you are aware of the dangers and do what is necessary to protect yourself from them, you can save yourself from illness and misery.

As a child growing up in rural Alabama it was common for people to die from encephalitis, which is transmitted when a mosquito carrying the parasite bites the victim. Once in the human body, the parasites travel to the brain, where they multiply until they cause the brain to swell and the victim to go insane before dying. An article in the Washington Post with the headline:

Mosquito Is Linked To Deadly Virus, Worrying Health Officials

---

[17]   © 1992 by The New York Times Company. Reprinted by permission.

Worm Uses Hormone Of the Immune System To Infect and Multiply

Scientists gain insight into a puzzling disease.

By GINA KOLATA

ONE of the great unsolved challenges of biology is to understand how they pairs of parasitic worms, which live their entire lives copulating in a blood vessel, manage to escape all the body's defenses.

The worms somehow know exactly where to settle in and start mating. The thousands of eggs they release each day are somehow walled off by the body in tiny granulomas, masses of white blood cells, where they are protected from the immune system and the body is protected from toxins in the eggs. The entire system seems incredibly complex and almost impenetrable.

The lives and survival strategies of the worms are of more than academic interest. The worms cause schistosomiasis, a parasitic disease that has persisted for centuries and that afflicts an estimated 200 million people today. Even though there is a drug, praziquantel, that can cure the disease, people can be reinfected. And some people die because the drug is not available in many isolated areas.

"It's a disease that has been very difficult to control," said Dr. Alan Sher, a schistosomiasis researcher at the National Institute of Allergy and Infectious Diseases.

Peeling Away Confusion

But now a group of researchers has, with a single stroke, peeled away layers of detail and confusion. They have revealed that at least one species of the worms, Schistosoma mansoni, appears to recruit exactly the immune system hormone that white blood cells release as part of an inflammatory response. And the researchers hypothesize, the worms then use the hormone, tumor necrosis factor, to find the blood vessel where they will live to stimulate themselves to produce eggs and to force the body to encase their eggs.

"The worm has evolved to use immune system signals," said Dr. James K. McKerrow the University of California in San Francisco. The finding, by Dr. McKerrow and his colleagues was published in a recent issue of Nature, a British science journal. Although parasitologists said the discovery did not immediately suggest a a better drug or a vaccine for the disease, it showed a new direction for research.

Dr. Sher said the finding was a surprise. He added that before this no one had any idea what signals the worms needed to lay eggs.

Dating to 2000 B.C.

The first written mention of schistosomiasis was in the time of the Egyptian pharaohs, around 2000 B.C. The disease was so common that infection with the parasite was considered a rite of passage and blood in the urine, a symptom of one form of schistosomiasis, was viewed as sign of puberty in boys.

Infected people excrete the microscopic, brownish-yellow eggs in their feces. If the eggs get into fresh water, the free swimming embryos escape, skittering about until they find a snail. They invade the snail and begin to multiply. Weeks later, thousands of larvae pour into the water.

When a person steps into the water the larvae rush over to burrow into the skin. From the skin, they enter the bloodstream and travel in it until they reach the lungs, where they stay for 10 days developing into white males and darker females. Then the worms re-enter the bloodstream. One species travels to the veins that drain the upper intestine, and another, Schistosoma mansoni, goes to those that drain the lower intestine. Worms of a third species go to veins that drain the bladder. There they stay, copulating for the rest of their lives, which may be 20 or 30 years.

Each pair of worms excretes thousands of eggs a day. About half of the eggs burrow through the walls of the intestine or bladder, depending on the species, and are excreted and continue the organism's life cycle. The others are swept in the blood to the liver, where they are encased in granulomas.

It is easy to spot a granuloma-infested liver, said Dr. S. Michael Phillips of the University of Pennsylvania Medical School. The granulomas dot the liver, looking like raised white bumps the size of a pinhead.

"The granuloma looks like a ball," Dr. Phillips said. "In the center of the ball is an egg, and around the eggs are immune system cells."

But one mystery of granulomas was what made them form. The egg lodges in the liver, stimulates T cells, white blood cells of the immune system, to swarm to the scene, and then, said Dr. Sher, the T cells "bring in a whole bunch of other cells, almost like a cascade." The entire system looked incredibly complex.

And a mystery of egg production was what signaled it. Researchers could isolate adult worms and maintain them, still coupled, in the laboratory, but they ceased to secrete eggs.

An answer arose when Dr. McKerrow and colleagues decided to study an observation made earlier by Dr. Sher others that no one had pursued. The researchers had been studying a strain of mice without an immune system to learn how it affected the development of schistosomiasis. They noticed that the mice never made granulomas. But, the researchers found, when they provided the mice with white blood cells, they suddenly began doing so.

At that point, said Dr. Richard M. Locksley, a member of the group who is an expert on immune system hormones, they decided to ask whether it was the hormones the cells secrete, known as cytokines, that allowed the worms to make eggs. They added cytokine after cytokine until they hit on tumor necrosis factor.

The researchers discovered that when they dripped tumor necrosis factor on worms in the laboratory they laid eggs. When they infused the factor into infected mice with no immune systems, the mice excreted eggs and formed granulomas.

Dr. Locksley said the findings suggest a coherent story of how the worms survive and thrive. It begins with bacteria, which inhabit the intestines. These bacteria normally have endotoxins, poisons that are trapped in their cell walls. When the bacteria die, these endotoxins are released into the vein that carries blood from the intestine to the liver.

Macrophages in the vein come upon the endotoxins, sense a bacterial attack, and secrete tumor necrosis factor. So, Dr. Locksley said, there is always some tumor necrosis factor floating in that particular vein but the cytokine is not normally present in any other blood vessel in the body.

At the start of an infection, meanwhile, worms leave the lungs and float through the blood, looking for their final home. When they come upon tumor necrosis factor in a blood vessel, they remain there. The nutrients being carried from the intestine to the liver feed them. And the tumor necrosis factor that is always present stimulates them to lay eggs.

worms to make eggs. They added cytokine after cytokine until they hit on tumor necrosis factor.

Some of those eggs float downstream to the liver. There, tumor necrosis factor is released by macrophages that creep through the tissue and initiate the formation of a granuloma. "Tumor necrosis factor recruits other cells and allows the granuloma to round off and get larger and wall off the egg," Dr. Locksley said.

As more and more eggs get encased in granulomas, the liver begins to swell and harden. Eventually, after many years, the liver function is severely impaired or destroyed. But Dr. Phillips cautioned that even if this description was correct in all details it was not yet clear how to use it to treat the disease. Although it might sound reasonable to give patients a drug that counteracts tumor necrosis factor, that could actually make matters worse, he said. The granulomas that eventually destroy the liver function also protect it from the worm's eggs. "Eggs make substances that damage the liver," he explained. So to live with the worm, he said, "what you want is a very close balance between just enough of a granuloma to protect against the eggs but not so much response that products of the granuloma becomes pathogenic."

Still, Dr. Sher said, there is something intellectually pleasing about cutting thorough so much of the confusion and showing, he said, "that a parasite might be using a cytokine for part of its biology."

Challenge: to battle a parasite without destroying the body's defenses.

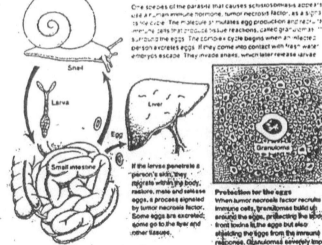
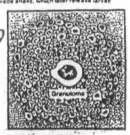

Parasitic Invader Uses Victim's Defenses

One species of the parasite that causes schistosomiasis appears to use a human immune hormone, tumor necrosis factor, as a signal in its life cycle. The molecule stimulates egg production and recruits immune cells that produce tissue reactions, called granulomas that surround the eggs. The complex cycle begins when an infected person excretes eggs. If they come into contact with fresh water embryos escape. They invade snails, which later release larvae

Snail

Larva

Liver

Egg

Small intestine

If the larvae penetrate a person's skin, they migrate within the body, mature, mate and release eggs, a process signaled by tumor necrosis factor. Some eggs are excreted; some go to the liver and other tissues.

Granuloma

Protection for the eggs
When tumor necrosis factor recruits immune cells, granulomas build up around the eggs, protecting the body front toxins in the eggs but also shielding the eggs from the immune response. Granulomas severely impair liver function.

Source: Nature; Edna McConnell Clark Foundation

One species of the parasite that causes schistosomiasis appears to use a human immune hormone tumor necrosis factor as a signal in its life cycle. The molecule stimulates egg production and recruits immune cells that produce tissue reactions, called granulomas that surround the eggs. The complex cycle begins when an infected person excretes eggs. If they come into contact with fresh water, embryos escape. They invade snails which later release larvae. If the larvae penetrate a person's skin, they migrate within the body, mature, mate and release eggs, a process signaled by tumor necrosis factor. Some eggs are excreted; some go to the liver and other tissues.

© 1992 by The New York Times Company. Reprinted by permission.

The article goes on to say:

"For the first time since the feared Asian tiger mosquito entered the continental United States in 1985, scientists have found it to be carrying a serious disease that could be transmitted to humans: Eastern equine encephalitis, a relatively rare but usually fatal brain affliction."[18]

Last summer in Maryland horses were found to be infected with Eastern equine encephalomyelitis, a form of encephalitis spread by mosquitoes. The Asian Tiger mosquito, which can transmit one of the more fatal forms of encephalitis, has been found in Alabama, Arkansas, Delaware, Florida, Georgia, Hawaii, Illinois, Indiana, Kansas, Kentucky, Louisiana, Maryland, Missouri, Mississippi, North Carolina, Ohio, Oklahoma, South Carolina, Tennessee, Texas and Virginia. Eighty percent of the people who contract the virus have their brains completely destroyed.

The mosquito has a white stripe down its back and white specks on its legs. Eating raw garlic everyday in summer will help keep mosquitos away. I have tried this and it works. They can't stand the smell as garlic permeates every cell of your body.

There is a plant that repels mosquitoes, a species of geranium called the Mosquito Plant. It is available at Michigan Bulb Company, Dept RK-13, 1950 Waldorf NW, Grand Rapids, Michigan 49550. Plant them around where you sit outside. They grow very large, and it is then that they effectively repel the pests.

Every year there are numerous cases of malaria reported in America, which had been completely eliminated at one point.

Optimism Dims In Effort On Malaria As It Spreads[19]

Southern Rose Cream effectively repels mosquitoes. You especially want to repel the mosquito carrying the dreaded West Nile virus.

---

[18]   © 1992 by The Washington Post, Washington, DC. Reprinted with permission.

[19]   © 1991 by The New York Times Company. Reprinted by permission.

While watching my ex-husband die from something that ate away his brain, I thought of all the times we went fishing together when he refused to use insect repellant. After our trips, he would have hundreds of mosquito bites on him. I am convinced that he died from some form of encephalitis, although the doctors did not seem to know exactly what was wrong, as the diagnosis kept changing.

While he was in the hospital, I had a few confrontations with nurses who tended the patient next to him, and then came over to attend to my ex, without changing their gloves. I had a fit! I let them have it each time, explaining the importance of not spreading disease. I find, again and again, articles like the one in The Washington Post with the headline:

Hand-Washing Practices A Problem
in Hospitals
A smaller headline read:
Fewer Than Half Comply, Study Shows.[20]

In the study, participants were informed that it was being conducted, yet 40 percent still did not comply with the requirement.

I observed that these germ theories clearly were correct, and changed my strategy for survival. People in my family called me rude because I left the room when a friend had a severe sneezing, coughing fit. (The same person later took a TB test that came up positive, so I'm glad I left.) But what about the people and children who stayed in the room while he was coughing?

Did you know that cattle often become infected with TB? There have been too many stories to ignore the possibility of cattle infected with TB being shipped to us in America from Mexico. In light of all the antibiotics, growth hormones and diseases that cows carry, I don't eat beef.

In the past the consensus has been that people need to know that they must cook the meat well enough to kill the germs, but do we want to eat beef with TB

---

[20]   © 1993 by The Washington Post, Washington, DC.

in it, whether it is dead or alive? I certainly don't like the idea of eating dead TB germs, dead E. Coli or scrapie, the mad cow encephalitis.

Trade Pact Raises Threat of TB From Cattle

"I am counsel, with the Government Accountability Project, to Wilfredo Rosario, a Department of Agriculture veterinary meat inspector who blew the whistle in 1990 on an illegal move by the department to allow beef containing laboratory-confirmed tuberculosis lesions approval as human food."

"Although most people cook their meat adequately to kill TB bacteria, it is reckless to dismiss cavalierly an unquantifiable health threat simply by stating that "veterinary officials are virtually unanimous in their opinion that bovine tuberculosis represents little threat to people." (Letter to the Editor from Ken Morrison, Los Angeles, Nov. 16, 1993)[21]

In reference to the last paragraph, what about those who eat "steak tartar," a dish consisting of raw ground beef?

Did you figure out yet why your six-year old has pubic hair and the first signs of breasts? When it happened with my six-year old and I took him to a doctor, I was told that it was because of the growth hormones in the milk and meat! I felt I had abused my child by giving him the adulterated foods!

Dangerous Hormone

"The Food and Drug Administration has approved injection of cow growth hormone, bovine somatotropine, in our country's cows to increase milk production as much as 20 percent. We don't allow our Olympic athletes to inject themselves with human growth hormone, yet we are allowing the food

---

[21]   © 1993 by The New York Times Company. Reprinted by permission.

supply to be contaminated by cow growth hormone." (Letter to the Editor by Gary Gibbs, New York, Nov. 9, 1993)[22]

"Massive overuse of antibiotics on the farm is breeding strains of drug-resistant microorganisms that make these medications worthless in fighting human disease."

© 1985 by Nutrition Action Healthletter published by The Center For Science in The Public Interest. 1875 Connecticut Avenue NW, Suite 300, Washington, DC 20009. Excerpt from original article entitled ANTIBIOTICS: SQUANDERING A MEDICAL MIRACLE is reprinted with permission.

Antibiotics In Feed Becoming Useless In Human Therapy

As if out of the minds of science fiction writers, certain infectious diseases-strains of meningitis, gonorrhea, salmonella, and others-are now becoming resistant to modern medicine's conventional means of treatment. These diseases, for decades under the control of physicians, have been accounted for innumerable deaths, many to children, because the illnesses did not succumb to the antibiotics which in the past were effective in killing the bacteria. Although there is considerable controversy over the source of this resistance, many scientists now believe that part of the population of resistant bacteria is originating from a seeming distant source: the use of antibiotics in animal feed.

According to scientists, a small minority of bacteria normally found in the intestines of animals and people is capable of warding off the toxic effect of antibiotics. When the drugs are taken into the body, however, they eliminate the bacteria still sensitive to antibiotics, which are normally in the vast majority; meanwhile, the resistant bacteria multiply.

This resistance to antibiotics, scientists are saying, is capable of being transferred from one bacterium to another in the animal's intestines and to bacteria in the environment-lakes, soil, air. Many scientists maintain that some of the bacteria that become resistant can cause diseases in humans.

© 1980 by Nutrition Action Healthletter published by The Center For Science in The Public Interest. 1875 Connecticut Avenue NW, Suite 300, Washington, DC 20009. Excerpt from original article reprinted with permission.

[22]   © 1993 by The New York Times Company. Reprinted by permission.

When a person sneezes, 600,000 germs are released into the air. They waft in the air for a minute because they are lighter than the air. Researchers have proved that the most likely way that you will catch a cold is to breathe in some of these 600,000 germs, or pick them up from a door knob or light switch and touch your eyes, nose, mouth or genitals while the germs are still alive. And some of them, especially some flu viruses, can make themselves dormant for four years, until they find a warm, moist host.

When you touch the contaminated surface and then touch your mucous membranes with your contaminated hand, you infect yourself with the germ, for these are passageways to your immune system. A simple environmental germ, once it makes its way into the vagina, causes Toxic Shock Syndrome, which is often fatal.

The message about the importance of hygiene has to be heard, yet 40 percent of health care workers still do not wash their hands before they touch a patient. I only had to look in my own office to see how disease spreads. Whenever someone was out with a cold or the flu, I began to notice a pattern of illness. It happened frequently that the replacement for the sick person soon fell ill after working at the person's work area.

Within a matter of days the new replacement fell ill. His or her replacement fell ill as well within a few days. Sometimes I'd watch three or four people come down sick. To test the germ theory, I sprayed the work area with hydrogen peroxide, an anti-infective, and the next person who filled in stayed healthy.

I often saw people who hung around together share illnesses. One would come down with a virus, and sure enough, the other soon followed. The simple fact is that when we sneeze, those 600,000 germs are released into the air. Catch them all in your hand? Impossible! Since most of them are lighter than air, they linger in the air awhile. This is one of the most common modes of transmission of infection.

And because I learned my lesson from these past experiences, and prefer to never take a chance on falling ill, I got in the habit of always sanitizing a new work area by simply spraying it with 3 percent hydrogen peroxide before using it. If there is a keyboard involved, spray the peroxide on a cloth and wipe it off.

There are some extremely toxic germs in our environment, particularly some influenza viruses. In some office environments I went into, there were "resident viruses" that the workers kept spreading among themselves. I rarely caught these viruses.

To save yourself from illness, here are some common overlooked instances of infection:

1. When sharing food, like at buffet-style dinners, do not touch the serving spoon to your plate. This can infect the serving spoon with germs that can be spread to others.
2. To prevent the above from happening, insist that everyone going back for seconds use a clean plate. The best restaurants do.
3. Don't share finger foods that sit and are refilled for each new customer. Why? The person who ate the nuts or pretzels before you got traces of his saliva on his hands, which gets on some of the nuts left in the dish when he reaches in for more. Do you really want to ingest that other person's saliva? In it will be anything infectious that he or she is carrying, and which could be passed on to you.
4. Don't share dips that people bite off of a chip or cracker and dip back into the dip.
5. Don't put the mouthpiece of your cigarette on the mouthpiece where 10 or 20 other smokers put their cigarettes in the course of that day or evening. Some of the things you can pick up: TB, herpes, hepatitis B and a host of other unwanted ailments.
6. Don't allow the water from the toilet to pop up on your genitals. The microbes in the toilet water can cause infections.
7. Amazingly, I have seen mothers take their nice clean babies and put him/her on someone's filthy floor. Then they wonder why the baby gets sick.
8. Avoid tight clothes, belts, socks, shoes, hair styles and jewelry. The interference of the natural flow of your bodily fluids can cause them to get stuck, putrefy and cause you pain and suffering. In addition, 10 years of tight socks can dangerously narrow blood vessels and impede proper blood flow.

For example, contrary to what has always been popular belief, that chills cause colds, studies done at Harvard and other reputable institutions have proved that people do not get viruses and germs unless exposed to them. I would like to interject that contrary to their findings, I believe that stress and getting chilled can also activate viruses that are dormant in the body and cause colds just as stress and illness can activate a dormant herpes virus.

Actually, our brains are designed to last longer than a lifetime, but our bodies usually wear out long before our brains are gone. Hopefully, we can change that by increasing awareness about health. Research has proved that:

●Tuberculosis, pneumonia, and whooping cough are only spread by direct contact with the germs. That means that someone with TB in the same room with you can infect you. This simple iota of information could save many people from contracting this dreaded disease.

●Tuberculosis, which had almost been eliminated in the United States, has made an unwelcome return. Worse, doctors are finding an alarmingly increasing number of people with drug-resistant TB. The scary thing about this highly contagious killer is that is can be transmitted simply from breathing the same air that an infected person breathes.

A slew of information about drug-resistant TB has poured out lately. This is a dreaded killer that causes much misery and pain.

TB, Easily Transmitted, Adds a Peril to Medicine appeared in The New York Times.

"First we had to deal with AIDS, now it's TB, and TB is a much bigger worry since it's transmitted through the air."[23]

The New York Times contained the following:

Top Scientists Warn Tuberculosis Could Become Major Threat

"The top Federal AIDS scientist, Dr. Anthony S. Fauci, raised the possibility today that the spread of drug-resistant tuberculosis might become as serious

---

[23]   © 1992 by The New York Times Company. Reprinted by permission.

a public health threat as AIDS unless a major new research effort was begun against tuberculosis."[24]

Agency Cites Urgent Need To Fight Increase In TB

"Tuberculosis will claim 30 million lives over the next 10 years unless more money is found to prevent its spread. The health agency declared tuberculosis a global emergency in April, noting that it killed more adults each year than all other infectious diseases combined. In the United States, 15 million people are infected."[25]

Obviously, this threat is real. Therefore, protect yourself from those who are infectious and being uncivil to expose the general public to their ills. Your body is what you experience life with. It is the only body that we know we have and we have a responsibility to keep it disease free so that we can experience a high quality of good health, and thus, life.

What about the old saying that "Oh what the heck, there are so many germs out there, we might as well get used to ingesting them in order to grow an immunity to them." It doesn't make sense that anyone would want to grow an immunity to a flu virus by catching it. Sure you get an immunity to that particular strain of the flu after you've caught it. The flu shot gives you the same immunity. Logically, it's better to avoid any virus.

> *Strengthening The*
> *Immune System*
> *Strengthens Life*

The final word is in and all the researchers have agreed on one thing: strengthening the immune system for short periods on a regular basis strengthens and prolongs life - - and improves the quality of a person's health and their ability

---

[24]   © 1992 by The New York Times Company. Reprinted by permission.

[25]   © 1992 by The New York Times Company. Reprinted by permission.

to fight diseases remarkably! The immune system can be strengthened in a number of ways: meditating, aerobic exercises, proper nutrition, proper breathing, homeopathic medicines, fresh air and sunlight, massage, swimming, jogging, and walking briskly are a few.

What ensues when it becomes activated is a cleansing and strengthening of your body. Your blood becomes oxygenated and toxins that have been building up in lymph fluids (you would know this as stiffness or soreness, like of the neck or shoulders) are moved into the blood. Anything that causes us to breathe deeply and fully for a sustained period, usually twenty minutes, oxygenates the body and stimulates the immune system, and it is then, like a furnace being turned on full blast, that it becomes fully activated.

These activities cause the brain to fill the body with endorphins (a hormone (peptide) of the brain with opiate-like and healing capabilities. If you want to have a psychic out-of-body experience, have a two hour acupressure massage. It will give you a natural high and change your consciousness to super relaxed and aware. Massage is an excellent way to strengthen your immune system, relax your body and expand your mind. It will immediately lower your blood pressure. An hour of massage has been proved to oxygenate the body as much as running for two miles.

> ## A Lot Of Things Weaken
> ## The Immune System

In 1984, the federal Centers For Disease Control estimated that 80,000 people a year were reported to die from eating from dirty hands. Considering that this is probably a small percentage of the actual amount, the ramifications of the actual figures would be staggering. Do you ever eat with your hands without washing them?

People can contract the famed British "mad cow" disease from handling infected sheep and not properly washing their hands, and from eating infected sheep or cow brains.

Spongiform or "mad-cow disease," also known as scrapie, is caused by a contagious microbe that goes to the person's brain and eats it away. Autopsies reveal that the brains of it's victims look like swiss cheese. It can be spread from eating the undercooked infected brain of a cow or sheep or handling an infected cow or sheep and not washing hands. There is a recipe that calls for cow or sheep brains to be sauteed lightly in onions and eggs. We ate them for many meals as a kid, but I would not touch them now.

The disease that can result from eating an infected brain is called Creutzfeldt-Jakob disorder when humans contract it. It is a form of encephalitis that is infectious and can be passed on genetically.

The following article discusses the disease, which has eluded scientists for a hundred years and is just coming to be understood.

HOW NOW, MAD COW?

Salmonella isn't the only risk of recycling animals into feed. For centuries sheep have suffered from scrapie, a disease that leaves their brains riddled with holes. But in 1986, scientists in England saw something new: cows started getting a similar disease, called bovine spongiform encephalopathy or BSE.

Researchers believe that cows get BSE when they eat animal feed that has been made from scrapie-infected sheep. A few years after being infected, the cows start to stagger and sometimes turn violent, which is how BSE acquired its nickname, "mad cow disease." BSE has struck more than 20,000 cows in Great Britain. Fortunately, no cases have yet been documented in the U.S.

When in Great Britain, play it safe by avoiding meat products that might contain brains (they have the highest levels of the BSE agent). That means sausages, pies, pates, canned meats or soups or entrees made with meat stock. Muscle (most meat) and milk have little or none of the BSE agent. Cooking doesn't affect the risk.

© 1992 by **Nutrition Action Healthletter,** published by The Center For Science In The Public Interest, 1875 Connecticut Avenue NW, Suite 300, Washington, DC 20009. Excerpt from original article reprinted with permission.

Your loving pets very often may be the cause of some of your illnesses. Part of the down side of being a pet owner is the array of diseases that come along with pets, some of which are:

- Cat scratch fever, which ranges from mild to severe and can cause brain swelling, encephalitis, seizures, coma and death;

We now know that Lyme disease is so impossible to avoid due to all the vectors that carry it, that everyone has it and needs to be detoxed of it.

- Rabies, which causes the brain to swell and is often fatal; .

- Flea bites, which can transmit viruses;

- Strep and coliform infections from dogs;

- Intestinal roundworm from dogs and cats; intestinal hookworm from dogs and cats;

- Toxoplasmosis from cats can cause birth defects and which more than 3,000 babies are born with each year;

- Ringworm, which is highly contagious and hard to eliminate;

- Scabies and Rosacea which come from a mite;

- Salmonella from lizards, eggs, chickens and turtles.

There is another way that we get diseases from pets that is still quite mysterious. When I was fourteen, a dear friend's mother fell ill. After many, many tests it was discovered that she had contracted a disease from kissing and eating after her French poodle that caused a parasite that lived in the dog's mouth to travel to her brain, where they hatched, and proceeded to crawl around on her brain and drive her insane.

It was a small town and everyone eventually found out everything about everyone else, and the word got out that my friend's mother died from a monstrous disease she got from eating after and kissing her pet.
Then in May of 1990, an article in The New York Times:

THE BACTERIA AT THE TABLE, which was about the twentieth such article I had read on food contamination, appeared. It sent me reeling to discover that according to an expert:

> "...*60 percent of everything in the retail case is contaminated*" and that "...*40 percent of our poultry is often contaminated*," and that "...*40,000 cases of salmonellosis were reported to the Centers for Disease Control in 1988, and this may be only 1 percent of all cases.*"[26]

What did I do after reading facts like the above in so many places? I sent copies to my mother and vowed to eat out less. I started to grow my own vegetables, which truly gives one a sense of why we need to wash raw foods in a safe antiseptic and rinse well before eating them.

> *We Must Not Forget The*
> *Basic Laws of Nature!*

In any situation, they are there whether we are ignorant of them or not. Therefore it is important that we know what they are. As you have learned, one of the important laws of nature is that germs and bacteria cause disease. A particularly nasty germ can be found in a particularly nasty place, in fecal matter. Fecal matter commonly and almost always contains *E. Coli*, an intestinal bacteria that is fatal to humans in small amounts.

---

[26]   © 1990 by The New York Times Company. Reprinted by permission.

I have bought bags of cow manure that had printed on the bag that it had been sterilized. Can this guarantee me that there is no E. Coli? It should. However, does a farmer who has two thousand cows sterilize his fertilizer before his uses it on the vegetables he grows and sells at the market?

I try to make sure most of what I eat is organic and these food are often grown with cow manure, which could contain E. Coli which can be especially fatal to children. I recommend to rinse filthy veggies in a salt water solution which will cause every drop of dirt to fall off, then soak immersed for minimum of 5 minutes in a solution of 1/2 cup of baking soda and ¼ cup 3% hydrogen peroxide to 1 quart of water. Then rinse with pure water. You can wash 3 heads of lettuce like this and drain them and wrap them in bundles in paper towels so you can cut up one when you want a salad. When you come back to get it you will find it fresher and more vibrant that it has been. It has soaked in some of the oxygen from the cleansing and a super lettuce.

Coming from a rural area in Alabama, I know what happens when you kill ten or twenty chickens at a time, or when any animal is slaughtered. It immediately loses control of its sphincter muscle and if they are all thrown into a large vat for cleaning, they most likely end up floating in a poop soup.

How much of that poop soup do you think is left on the chicken when you get it from the market? Some people rinse their chickens in a solution of clorox water. I would not want to eat chicken with a thin film of clorox water or a thin film of poop either.

Even a thin film of poop could be dangerous if you threw the chicken on the grill for three minutes on each side. Any meat I eat gets washed first in a solution of peroxide or vinegar, unless I get it at the Amish Farmers Market at Rt. 29 and Rt. 198 in Burtonsville, Maryland and it has been cooked. This does not mean that they all do it, but I spoke to an Amish farmer once who said he fed his chickens hydrogen peroxide because it made them hardier, he lost less of them, and they got sick less often.

Since 70 percent of what I eat is raw, it is critical that the food be uncontaminated. It is my responsibility and mine alone that I render it uncontaminated before it enters my body. Since I started living this way I rarely get sick anymore and I love it. Life feels great when you are at maximum health. The washes described above for fruits and vegetables effectively eliminate harmful germs and bacteria that get on our food from the environment, for the oxygen, salt and vinegar neutralizes them.

Another basic law of nature: we are all seriously affected by toxins and pathogens in our food. This means we must be responsible for what goes into our bodies. It is the only vehicle we have to take us through this life.

At times when a problem in the food industry is exposed, there begins a tide of activity by various groups in trying to solve it. Horror stories have abounded for the last hundred years, with problems ranging from salmonella in chickens, meats, and eggs to flu viruses in chickens to selenium overdoses in chickens, with no end in sight.

Sometimes when I speak to a stranger about sources of contamination in America like: contaminated seafood, malaria, mosquitos that can give a fatal encephalitis, that there are 439,999 abandoned toxic waste dumps in America, the hazards of chlorine, insidious parasites that are commonly found in dirt everywhere that bore through our skin and live off of our bodies, I am amazed to hear the person say, "Our government would not allow us to be exposed to such widespread contamination." I am mentioning it here because I have gotten so many similar responses from so many people.

My regret for them is that they do not know and they do not seem to want to know. The most terrible thing about living with pollution and hazardous conditions is being ignorant of how much they are harming you and doing nothing about it until you discover you and your kids got cancer from the toxic waste dump you've been living on top of. The only good thing about this entire situation is our becoming aware of it so we can stop it.

> # Being Aware Of
> # Contamination Can Save
> # You

In addition to the following sources of environmental contamination, there are many others, and sometimes they can not be avoided. Some of the more common ones are:

- Gas fumes
- Food preservatives, colorings, pesticides
- Smog, chemical fumes
- Nylon, synthetic fibers
- Floor polishes, after shaves, hair sprays
- The propellant in aerosol sprays and other hydrocarbons

What do you do when someone spills chlorine (yes, plain laundry bleach, one of the most carcinogenic substances known to man), in your office? You either leave until someone cleans up the spill, or you clean it up yourself. No, you should not stay there and ignore it.

If you are pregnant then you had better get out of there quickly! The fumes can cause brain damage and other serious damage to your body and cells, and nervous system. Fetuses are especially vulnerable.

If pregnant don't sniff, don't even let a whiff of chlorine near you. Although you will want to avoid chlorine even if you are not pregnant, for even the fumes can do you in. Chlorine is absorbed into the bloodstream through the skin. The fumes are more toxic to the lungs and respiratory system than the chlorine that is absorbed into the bloodstream when chlorine touches the skin.

If you spilled chlorine in a large area, you would want to ventilate and leave the area for as long as possible to allow some of the fumes to dissipate. Use rubber gloves if you must touch it at all and long handled utensils to remove it. A fan taking the fumes away from you is preferable to opening a window and having no extraneous ventilation. Yet how many people are still sticking their bare hands in clorox solutions everyday? Worse, how many children?

What about the chlorine in scouring powder? Yes, it is toxic as well so use a brush or rubber gloves when using it. Do not touch it with your bare hands. Think of all the damaged children who got that way from their mothers not knowing the danger of using heavy solutions of chlorine all their young lives. There is one good thing about chlorine, it is a strong antiseptic agent capable of killing the most resistant bacteria and viruses, even the AIDS virus.

Is it a myth that it is safe to drink after someone if what you are drinking contains alcohol, since liquor is supposed to kill germs? I've heard many people say alcohol kills germs. The truth is that alcohol is a mild antiseptic that will reduce the chances of disease being spread, however, it is not a total antiseptic and will not prevent the spread of colds and sore throats. Under an article called

Germs In The Chalice

". . .Dr. Giordano said, he would warn patients with colds or sore throats not to share any drinking vessel, including a communion chalice."[27]

> *How Did So Many*
> *People Who Never*
> *Smoked Get Cancer?*

Ever wonder how so many people who never smoked got lung cancer? Everyday when we shower we are exposing ourselves to the chlorine in the water fumes, which is four times more toxic than chlorine is on the skin. Fortunately, it is

---

[27]   © 1991 by The New York Times Company. Reprinted by permission.

diluted in the water. To minimize the risks, ventilate the shower, and don't make the water too hot. If possible, open a window. Try to keep your back to the shower while leaving the shower curtain open enough for ventilation to occur.

Many people got lung cancer from industrial contamination. For many years people were not aware of the dangers of asbestos and it used to be used routinely dozens of times daily in the environment and handled unsafely (in flooring, roofing, shingles, insulation). How many people got cancer from asbestos?

Radon has been blamed for a long time for lung cancer in nonsmokers. Chlorine in the shower, in the coffee, dioxin in the white coffee filters, in the water, have been blamed! Microwaves, electromagnetic fields, industrial contamination and routine crop dusting with toxic pesticides have been blamed. Stress, smoking, drug abuse, ingesting toxins, especially lead, from fumes and in the drinking water have all been implicated for environmental carcinogenic contamination.

Report Ties Electrical Fields To Cancer

read the headline in a December 15, 1990 article in The New York Times.

"The strongest evidence of any link has come from studies in children, today's report said. Nine studies 'have consistently found modestly elevated risks (some statistically significant) of leukemia, cancer of the nervous system, and to a lesser extent, lymphomas,' it said."[28]

The Environmental Protection Agency has declared that electromagnetic fields from power lines and appliances can cause cancer. Prolonged exposure to them promotes the proliferation of cancer cells, suppresses immune function and the secretion of melatonin (a pineal hormone), which protects against breast and other cancers.

I am so sensitive to electromagnetic fields that I cannot stand to be in a room where a radio or TV is operating for more than five or ten minutes. I start to squint my eyes and grit my teeth, for the high pitched noise seems to be bouncing off my brain, and it hurts.

---

[28]   © 1990 by The New York Times Company. Reprinted by permission.

Since light suppresses melatonin secretion, sleep in a dark room. Melatonin has been proved to protect against malignant melanoma and other cancers.

If you have a history of breast cancer in your family, you can greatly improve your chances by eating lots of raw and cooked carrots for the beta carotene and taking 3-20 mg. of melatonin at bedtime. Too many studies have shown that heavy smokers who eat lots of beta carotene never get cancer whereas those with low beta carotene levels most certainly almost always get lung cancer.

This is vitally important information that every smoker needs to know. If you think about what this study means, doesn't it suggest that lung cancer in smokers is caused by a lack of beta carotene, and is therefore, a deficiency disease?[29] I think it does.

There is purportedly, however, a discrepancy as one study reported by CNN on April 13, 1994 claimed that 20 percent of those taking high doses of beta carotene were 18 percent more likely to develop cancer. I think that common sense should tell us that eating carrots raw or cooked is good for us.

I don't condone smoking, but here is a tip to minimize the damage you are doing by smoking. Do not breathe the smoke in so deeply. Make a conscious effort to take in half as much smoke as you have in the past. Doing this can effectively cut your damage in half.

With this new awareness about how our bodies may have been being polluted without our knowledge, we should, therefore, limit the number of toxins we take in by refraining from eating impure foods, reacquaint ourselves with healthy eating habits, and remove the toxins that we have ingested in the past.

Everyday we face a wide variety of cancer-causing agents in our environment without being aware of it. One of the least suspected is tap water, which studies say increase the risk of rectal and bladder cancer by 50 percent and raise the risk of other cancers as well. It is sometimes impossible to avoid these kinds of environmental pollutants, but you can strengthen your body so that their effect is minimized.

---

[29]   © 1993 by Life Extension Foundation, PO Box 229120, Hollywood, FL 33022-9120. 1-800-841-5433. Reprinted with permission.

Detox tea, found at any health food store, is helpful periodically. Fasting,[30] taking oxygen, getting the proper amount of exercise, eating correctly, making sure your body gets the minimum basic trace elements and maintaining proper fluid intake, which are all discussed in this book, will help in the detox process. Once every month or bimonthly clean out your colon.

No matter how well you eat, toxins accumulate in it. Herbs and natural substances are preferred to drugs for cleansing it. .

Two Healing Machines: Family Must-Haves For Health And Healing Crisis

These two machines can be used periodically for general health, and daily for a health crisis, like a severe diagnosis of any kind. Read what the manufacturers say:

1. **PYRO-ENERGEN produces and utilizes negatively-charged static electricity and has been proven to eradicate the root cause of various diseases such as HIV/AIDS, cancer, herpes, hepatitis, and influenza.** Static electricity exists naturally in our atmosphere and is essential to living things and beneficial to repel the world's maladies, thus, there are no side effects at all. Static electricity is therefore one of the best elements for the treatment of diseases.

PYRO-ENERGEN is the first and only one of its kind in the world. Other existing electrotherapy devices such as high voltage therapy machines and low voltage frequency generators induce current to our bodies. These machines produce man-made electricity that gives harmful side effects for humans! This company has agreed to give anyone who mentions that they heard about it from me $50 off on this machine. In order to get the discount, you need to call them to place your order. If you have someone direly ill, call me and get this machine. It is also good for the entire family's health.

https://www.pyroenergen.com/about.htm

---

[30]   I recommend one or two day fasts, with consumption of water and liquids such as organic apple juice, or any fruit juices and vegetable juices along with detox tea. Meditation, massage and participating in other measures for increasing your awareness are also helpful.

2. **Mesotherapy Needle-Free Silver Skin Rejuvenator. Use to massage the Rose cream in skin. I have found unbelievable ways to use this item that I will share with you.**
This one is a cellular cleanser that cleanses the Lymphatic system and the blood and promises to remove all scars. It actually burns up parasites using electrified silver and tourmaline using a safe mesotherapy process. Mesotherapy normally uses needles to implant medicines into the skin, however, this machine does it without needles. It works like nothing I have seen and I recommend use it with the Rose cream mixed with the one they provide for maximum cellular cleansing. It truly cleanses the lymphatic system and blood as well as kills parasites. These sell out quickly, they can barely cover the demand for them so get yours here while they last at this dirt cheap price. Others sell same machine for $1200-$3500 and this one is only $35. God led me to this one. **CAUTION**: The recommended dosage is 15 minutes a day. This machine is so powerful, I recommend only 5 minutes a day and you will experience amazing results. Use only for 1 minute on each problem. Overusing it longer than 5 minutes causes my body to feel super hot on the treated spots. I realized that it was the the result of the machine burning up toxins. I drank lots of Hydrogen/Oxygen water and quickly recovered. *If you need these machines in a crisis, then you need me. I am available for consultations for those who want my help.*

Everyone is being eaten alive by parasites. People have no idea what is living inside them. I have met thousands of people who thought they were clean because they did saunas, yoga, meditation, massage, neutraceuticals, doctors, microbiologists, teachers, people from all walks of life who were not awestruck and bewildered when the saw all the pounds of parasites come out of their bodies. Miraculously, weight fell off. These were the lucky ones. Everyone else will be slowly and meticulously eaten alive by parasites. My protocol, which uses the teachings of Jesus Christ, is the only comprehensive organic program that exists. And it only takes 5 minutes a day. This is the secret to eternal youth and beauty. No matter how well you eat or how much you exercise or soak out your pores in a spa, none of that will save you from the insidious parasites that eat everyone alive.

https://www.ebay.com/itm/Mesotherapy-Needlefree-Skin-Rejuvenation-Silver-Massage-Device-Anti-Age-Cream-/322625561017? trksid=p2141725.m3641.l6368

Don't want to take my word for it? Then all you have to do it so your own research and if you type into your browser, Do parasites eat everyone alive? and 260,000 websites come up telling you that yes, they do. Then go to youtube.com and type in *Monsters Inside Me*, to find the dozens of videos done by the Discovery Channel on how parasites eat us alive and parasites are usually the last thing people think is wrong with them. In my experience, it is parasites 99.9% of the time. Yet you will never see a parasite until you start killing them.
https://www.youtube.com/results?search_query=monsters+inside+me

Then search for The Body Snatchers by National Geographic and another slew of videos come up telling us that parasites are eating us alive.
https://www.youtube.com/results?
search_query=the+body+snatchers+by+national+geographic

Check out these worthwhile organizations:
National Liberty Alliance
   https://www.nationallibertyalliance.org/takebacktherepublic

 The mission of NLA is to restore the Republic and the Common Law courts which are Courts of Record, that is, restore the Constitution to the Supreme Law of the Land. This will restore and protect our unalienable rights. This is their Healing Call which is on Thursdays 8pm EST.
   https://www.nationallibertyalliance.org/natural%20healing%20call

The Real Truth Universe   **https://www.realtruthuniverse.com/home**
Fascinating information on a variety of topics and insider information. Very informative and highly recommended. Dr WC is informed and a highly valuable asset for those seeking knowledge. There is something for everyone here including me appearing monthly with timely health info to keep us healthy. https://www.realtruthuniverse.com/archives-2017

If you live in another county, check with your local health department for a similar service. In most states, free anonymous HIV screening as well as venereal disease screening are available.

A Hidden Source Of Contamination

Everything coming into the house gets wiped off or sprayed with 50% diluted Natural Herbal Lotion. Bags get sprayed and folded for recycling then placed in a sealed bag. Bedbugs and tiny creatures can come into your home from bags. How many hands have your items been through before they got to you? It's very hard to find anything in our society that did not come from China. Some of them were assembled by young people sitting on their lawn. In doubt? Start wiping off the things that come into your house from stores and shopping online. You will be amazed at the dirt. Which translates to microbes and disease for those unknowingly touching these contaminated items. The mail is filthy as it has been through 100-year old holding tanks that never get cleaned. People from all walks of life like the teenagers I met in the metro while in Paris who had dug out a home for themselves under an abandoned building are handling you items. Their floor, walls and ceiling was dirt. They had a baby and had high hopes of starting a band. They also assembled items they got from China and resold them on the street because they were not able to get papers to get a proper job because they were not French.

Chapter 15

> # *THERE ARE SOME GOOD BACTERIA*

There are some good bacteria that you will always want to have in your body, and they are the living ingredients found in yogurt, *Lactobacillus acidophilus, Lactobacillus bulgarius, Lactobacillus caucasicus* and other friendly flora that occur naturally in our bodies to help keep it healthy. You can find them in the dairy case at health food stores and some supermarkets. It is common knowledge that the Swiss live longer than we do because they ingest larger amounts of yogurt, which contains these essential good bacteria.

During the last few decades, levels of yeast in Americans have increased dramatically as a result of our over-processed modern diet. Drugs that kill off all bacteria in the body can have devastating consequences on a person's immune system. The result is Americans with less effective and efficient immune systems, for no longer are the good bacteria that keep us healthy present. Americans are learning, and we are wise to increase our consumption of yogurt, a natural immune-system booster.

Acidophilus (*Lactobacillus Acidophilus*)

It has been established that one important factor that contributes to good health is the number of friendly bacteria in our intestinal tract since they act as an antibiotic and crowd out candida and other pathogens. Acidophilus helps digestion, the absorption of vitamins and minerals, reduce cholesterol, the balance of intestinal flora and the making of B vitamins. Poor diet, antibiotics, toxins in foods, water and air reduces friendly flora in the intestine which can lead to gas, constipation and improper absorption of essential nutrients. An improper balance of intestinal flora could lead to an overgrowth of Candida, a harmless parasite that can wreak havoc on health if it gets out of control. In this aspect, acidophilus acts as an antibiotic as it binds with harmful substances and helps aid their excretion.

It can be purchased in capsules or found in acidophilus milk, yogurt, kefir and cheese.

Another immune system booster that is becoming famous, but which had been famous to the Chinese for centuries, is garlic. I casually recommended it as an immune system booster to a woman who complained that she was sick all the time with colds and viruses.

I saw her again a year later and she thanked me and hugged me and said her husband was so grateful to me for recommending the garlic. In fact she said he prepared it for her because he liked the way it kept her well. She said every week he presses a lot of garlic for her and mixes it with olive oil and they keep it in a jar in the refrigerator.

She adds it to her dinner salad every evening. According to her, taking garlic has made her well for the longest stretch of time than she has ever been well in her life!

Garlic has been known to cure several types of cancer and to prevent and help reverse heart disease. It is good for radiation and cell damage, and prevents premature aging. It helps prevent atherosclerosis, heart attacks and strokes. Garlic has over 100 sulphur-containing compounds, which act as an antibiotic in the body. Eat garlic everyday during the summer to keep mosquitoes away. It was put in a test tube with 28 cancer-causing substances and it wiped out every one of them. That's a lot of power in a little bulb! It's like a vitamin pill all by itself.

Probiotics Are The Good Bacteria That Make Immunity Stronger

I urge you go to these links and read. This stuff really turns on the immune system and does so much more. Mimi is great and very knowledgeable. This is the best probiotic I have found.

http://www.bravocoop.com/

http://www.bravocoop.com/#!The-Flutter-and-the-Shimmer-The-new-health-super-power/g8zu7/5650b47c0cf29d581a42b482

The following is excerpted from A CLOVE A DAY from Nutrition Action Healthletter, published by The Center For Science In The Public Interest at 1875 Connecticut Avenue NW, Suite 300, Washington, DC 20009. ℗ December, 1989. Article by Jayne Hurley and Stephen Schmidt.

A CLOVE A DAY?

"But for its odour," wrote Charak, the father of Hindu medicine, it "would be costlier than gold." Hippocrates used it to treat people for pneumonia and infected wounds. In 1858, Louis Pasteur announced that it killed bacteria.

During World War I it was rubbed on wounds to prevent gangrene. During World War II it was called "Russian penicillin."

Today, it is used by millions of people to treat everything from baldness to athlete's foot. But just tell your doctor you want to eat garlic to help keep your heart healthy or protect you from cancer, and you'll get either a shrug or a stern lecture about the folly of folk medicine.

Research is beginning to show that Charak and the others may have known whereof they spoke.

CLOVES AGAINST CHOLESTEROL

Is garlic good for our hearts? It's too early to tell for sure, but preliminary studies in animals and humans hint that garlic may lower levels of artery-clogging fats like LDL ("bad") cholesterol, and raise HDL ("good") cholesterol.

Garlic may help prevent heart disease in other ways, too. It appears to lengthen the time it takes blood to clot, and may actually help dissolve clots. (Most heart attacks and strokes occur when blood clots get stuck in narrowed arteries.)

Scientists have a clearer picture of garlic's effect on animals than on humans. When they fed raw garlic or garlic oil to rabbits and rats, LDL cholesterol dropped and HDL rose. But the amounts were equivalent to 14 to 230 cloves per day for a human. Garlic also seemed to prevent- and even reverse- the early stages of atherosclerosis.

When researchers fed rabbits a cholesterol-raising diet for three months, fatty plaque deposited on their arteries. Nine months later, animals that were given 1 to 1 and a half mg of garlic oil in their daily chow had fewer than half as many deposits as rabbits that received no garlic.

THE HUMAN CONDITION

Most studies in which people were fed large quantities of garlic show the same results: decreases in total cholesterol and LDL levels.

NATURE'S PENICILLIN

Though people have used garlic as a natural antibiotic for centuries, it's in the lab where garlic's anti-microbial properties have been most clearly observed.

It inhibits the growth of or kills two dozen kinds of bacteria (including Staphylococcus and Salmonella) and at least 60 types of fungi and yeast. The hero appears to be allicin, the chemical that's responsible for garlic's smell. so if you destroy the aroma-by cooking or processing-garlic may lose its ability to battle microbes.

During the days before synthetic antibiotics, garlic was often used to fight tuberculosis. Recently, Edward Delaha and Vincent Garagusi, of Georgetown University Hospital set out to confirm garlic's ability to kill tuberculosis and similar microbes, known as mycobacteria.

They added an allicin-rich garlic extract to 30 strains of mycobacteria growing in test tubes. A month later, the garlic had done critical damage to all 30.

Garagusi says he has approached several pharmaceutical companies with his findings, but that he has been unable to drum up any interest in garlic "therapy."

GARLIC AGAINST CANCER

Garlic may protect against cancer-at least in laboratory animals.

In an experiment by michael J. Wangovich, of Houston's M.D. Anderson Hospital, mice that were fed a component of garlic (diallyl sulfide) before being exposed to a cancer-causing chemical had 74 percent fewer colon cancer tumors than mice that received no garlic.

Wargovich speculates that large quantities of dialyl sulfide could help the liver detoxify the carcinogen.

Other animal studies show that garlic's sulfide conpounds can inhibit the development of cancer of the lung, large bowel, and esophagus.

"The National Cancer Institute is looking at ten compounds that are dynamite in preventing cancer in animal studies," says Wargovich.

If the NCI determines that the compounds are safe, the next step would be to study their effects in humans. And if those studies are positive, Wargovich says the food industry could fortify products with the compounds. "We'd have designer foods that help prevent cancer," he says.

Serrapeptase natural Cardiovascular cleanser eats up tumors, inflammation, cancer, cellular debris, blockages, blood clots, cleanses the body. Works better than one aspirin a day and is safer. Best to get proper dosing for your situation.

Liposomal Glutathione (GSH) is a protein naturally produced in every cell of our bodies known as a petide that is made up of cysteine, glutamine and glycine. Our bodies uses glutathione to protect us from the effects of physical and emotional stress, pathogens, toxins, free-radicals and aging. We find the highest concentration of this protein in our liver which cleans toxins from our bodies. It is a special antioxidant as it is the only one that can work with enzymes such as glutathione peroxidase to prevent oxidization of membranes. It also helps activate vitamin E and vitamin C and is credited with imparting longevity and health.

Studies have shown that cayenne not only boosts the immune system but removes the placque that builds up in arteriosclerosis. Studies have repeatedly proved that beta carotene not only boosts the immune system but prevents cancer and a number of other ills.

Vitamin A has proved to help prevent infections. Vitamin C is essential for hundreds of bodily functions, but particularly the immune system. Vitamin E stimulates the immune system and helps in detoxification and repair. Acidophilus and garlic strengthen the immune system.

Eating mostly fruits and vegetables stimulates the immune system because they impart essential disease-fighting ingredients into the body. For specific foods for certain illnesses, see the charts of natural and homeopathic remedies in Chapter 22.

Black Walnut

Is an herb that should not be taken if any chronic disease is present. It is good for eliminating the parasites that 90 percent of the population picks up commonly from municipal water supplies and going barefoot. Black Walnut and Bladderwrack cleanse the body of parasites and tapeworms. Black Walnut is also used in the treatment of lung diseases, tuberculosis, healing of sores of the mouth and throat.

Coenzyme Q_{10}

Coenzyme Q_{10} (ubiquinone), also known as CoQ is used by millions of people as a cancer fighter. It acts as a vitamin and declines in the body as it ages. It is an extremely vital catalyst in helping cells create the energy they need for life. It is present in all human systems and most human cells. In Japan 250 CoQs are made by 80 companies! It boosts immunity and overall health and is believed to be a more powerful antioxidant than vitamin E. It won't allow free radicals to accumulate. It boosts the immune system, strengthens the heart and extends life. As we age, we lose our ability to make it from other enzymes. Reduced levels lead to lower cell energy and lowered resistance to disease. It is crucial for aging and remaining ageless. It is used to treat and prevent aging, boost the immune system, protect the stomach lining and heal ulcers, dissolve tumors, treat leukemia, high blood pressure and heart disease. It has been shown to relieve asthma, allergies, brain abnormalities, obesity, candidiasis, MS, cancer, gum disease and diabetes. It should be bright yellow and has a short shelf life. It is abundant in salmon, sardines and mackerel.

Dandelion

A bitter herb that cleanses the blood and liver and, thus, stimulates the immune system. It is often used as a diuretic, but also improves pancreatic function, the spleen, stomach and kidneys. It is good for anemia, gout, jaundice, abscesses, boils, rheumatism, cramps, constipation and increasing the production of bile. It helps prevent cancer, especially of the breast, and reduces cholesterol and uric acid.

Echinacea (purple cone flour or thistle)

This is one of the bitter herbs. Traditionally is has been used by millions to prevent bacterial infections. It stimulates the immune system and detoxifies by pulling wastes out of lymph glands. It is good for colic, colds, flu, infections, and purifying the blood. Native Americans have long used it for snake bites. It is an antibiotic, antiviral and anti-inflammatory. It is good for swollen glands and has been known to eliminate tumors. Make sure you get the real thing, as there as been much deception with this herb. The freeze-dried variety is preferred. Smile Herb Shop in College Park, Maryland has an organic Echinacea.

Shiitake

Shiitake is the name for a famous healing Japanese mushroom that is used to treat cancer, high blood pressure, prevent aging, cholesterol and to increase energy. They are considered by the Chinese an exceptionally effective cure-all. They strengthen the immune system by producing interferon and eliminate a host of diseases.

Reishi is another type of shiitake mushroom. There are six types of reishi. They have been used for 2,000 years for their youth-giving properties and to promote vitality. These mushrooms are delicious in foods and should be eaten routinely for their protective effect. Add them to casseroles, gravies, sauces and stews.

Spirulina

Spirulina is a protein-rich algae that reduces both total cholesterol and LDL levels. Nutritionally, nothing else can compare to it. It is a complete food that contains essential fatty acids (gammalinolenic acid (GLA)) in abundance. GLA is the same immune system booster found in evening primrose oil and borage oil. It greatly enhances nutrient absorption from the small intestine into the blood stream and contains twenty times as much protein as soybeans (which have impressive amounts of protein), an ample amount of B_{12}, high iron, amino acids, beta carotene, enzymes, coenzymes, chlorophyll and the blue-green pigment phycocyanin which was found to extend the life of animals injected with cancer cells.

It contains four color pigments that have documented benefits as cancer preventatives. They are: chlorophyll, (green) phycocyanin (green precursor to chlorophyll), porphyrin (red pigment), and yellow pigments, which includes large amounts of beta carotene. All the color pigments have enzymes, coenzymes and other cancer-prevention nutrients.

Spirulina is good for fasting, mineral assimilation and nurturing the body. It us recommended especially for alcoholics and hypoglycemics.

I recently tested several spirulina's and all came back containing mold and parasites. I can no longer recommend it.

Royal Jelly Is King

The health benefits of royal jelly include it's ability to prevent certain types of cancers, lower blood pressure, treat sexual infertility, lower cholesterol levels, protect the liver, reduce inflammation, heal digestive disorders, prevent premature aging, help in weight loss, and increase circulation. It is used largely to strengthen immunity and help with conception

Chapter 16

DID WE REALLY DO ALL THAT DAMAGE TO OUR PLANET?

Unfortunately we did and still do!

The human race has been heavily polluting our earth's oceans, rivers, streams and wetlands for the past hundred years. The fish and crustaceans have no way to escape the contamination. It is not uncommon now that people become very ill and some even die after eating contaminated seafood. These are some of the reasons I have almost eliminated seafood from my diet with deep regret.

I love seafood. Lobster with drawn butter sauce is one of my favorites. I used to have it for breakfast. Alas, this desperate act comes only after reading countless, countless articles like the following on seafood contamination and feeling sick almost every time after eating seafood. Many people don't realize that their illness may have been caused by the seafood they ate hours before or at last night's dinner. It was difficult to give up a lifelong passion, but my health comes first.

It only makes sense if we sit down and think about it; it is impossible that the fish and flora can be unaffected by the toxic substances we dump into the waters they live in. These toxins are absorbed by them since they have no way to escape.

I have read the horror stories about people getting hepatitis from eating contaminated seafood and dying, or eating seafood from polluted waters and becoming severely ill. Coming from a long line of seafood lovers, I became acquainted with the hazards twenty years ago when my aunt got food poisoning from some fresh fried undercooked clams.

Following are only a few of the big time disasters that plague our environment and which every man, woman and child on earth is paying for because we are living with the pollution from them. These and hundreds of others

like them have made me cautious about eating anything that cannot escape the
polluted waterways of our world:

Leaking Tanks Pose Risks, Raise Cleanup Costs For Area Residents[31]

The Oozing of America
"The underground lake of petroleum now seeping into a Fairfax County
neighborhood 15 miles from Capitol Hill is only one of thousands of such
leaks across the nation in recent years."[32]

Top Worry: A Waste Tank That Belches
"Tank 101-SY is a million-gallon underground caldron of radioactive sludge
and toxic solvents and who knows what else, seething and brewing beneath
a semisolid crust that has formed atop the liquid"[33]

Tank Leaks Pose Risk, Raise Costs
Underground Woes Bubbling To Surface Across The Region.
"Thousands of aging underground tanks are leaking gasoline, heating oil and
other chemicals into the Washington region's environment, forcing residents
to find new water supplies. . ."[34]

---

[31]   © 1992 by The Washington Post, Washington, DC. Reprinted with permission.

[32]   © 1991 by The Washington Post, Washington, DC. Reprinted with permission.

[33]   © 1991 by The Washington Post, Washington, DC. Reprinted with permission.

[34]   © 1992 by The Washington Post, Washington, DC. Reprinted with permission.

Hanford Site Cleanup Seen As Daunting Task[35]

Hudson PCB Removal Stalled Again[36]

Estimates of Weapons Cleanup Inflated[37]

2 Admit EPA Violated Hazardous Waste Law In Issuing Permit
Regulators are termed too cozy with industry[38]

Uranium Dust At Ohio Plant Is Rated As High[39]

Radiation Effect Played Down At Uranium Plant[40]

Facing a Nightmare of Poisoned Earth

**Fukushima Is Continually Blasting All Of Us With High
Levels Of Cesium, Strontium And Plutonium And Will Slowly
Kill Millions For Years To Come. *This is the end of the
American Dream.***

http://endoftheamericandream.com/

http://endoftheamericandream.com/archives/fukushima-is-continually-
blasting-all-of-us-with-high-levels-of-cesium-strontium-and-plutonium-and-
will-slowly-kill-millions-for-years-to-come

Shipments of Seaweed Resume From Japan, The Most Irradiated Place
In The World
http://www.bing.com/videos/search?
q=latest+news+on+fukushima&&view=detail&mid=65179903B711B9A16983651
79903B711B9A16983&&FORM=VDRVRV

[37]   © 1991 by The New York Times Company. Reprinted by permission.

[40]   © 1991 by The Washington Post, Washington, DC. Reprinted with permission.

"...the most optimistic forecasts say it will take at least 30 years and 30 billion dollars to clean it up.[41]

Hanford Cleanup Could Cost 57 Billion[42]

Anger Lingers After Leak At Atomic Site[43]

2 Women At Rocky Flats Plant Tell Of Intimidation, Safety Violations[44]

E.P.A Urged To Ease Rules On Cleanup Of Toxic Waste
"Lower Standards And Fewer Safeguards"[45]

G.A.O. Urges Suspension Of New Pesticide-Testing Program
"The Government's newest program for testing pesticide residues in fruits and vegetables is unreliable and should be suspended, Congressional investigators say."[46]

---

[41]   © 1991 by The Washington Post, Washington, DC. Reprinted with permission.

[42]   © 1992 by The New York Times Company. Reprinted by permission.

[43]   © 1992 by The New York Times Company. Reprinted by permission.

[44]   © 1991 by The Washington Post, Washington, DC. Reprinted with permission.

[45]   © 1992 by The New York Times Company. Reprinted by permission.

[46]   © 1992 by The New York Times Company. Reprinted by permission.

Court Affirms Ban On Carcinogenic Pesticides In Processed Foods[47]

Appeals Court Strikes Down OSHA Standards On Toxic Exposure[48]

Russians Describe Dumping Of Nuclear Waste

"Worldwide Nuclear Waste Dumping, 4,977,028 curies"[49]

Toxic Agents Found To Be Killing
Off Whales

"Heavy concentrations of pollutants are found in beluga whales that die in St. Lawrence River"[50]

Spill Is A Sign Of Wider
Sewage Problems

"In a 1989 publication, The Natural Resources Defense Council estimated that 5 trillion gallons of industrial waste water and 2.3 trillion gallons of sewage- in various degrees of treatment- are released into America's coastal waters

---

[47]   © 1992 by The Washington Post, Washington, DC. Reprinted with permission.

[48]   © 1992 by The Washington Post, Washington, DC. Reprinted with permission.

[49]   © 1993 by The New York Times Company. Reprinted by permission.

[50]   © 1992 by The New York Times Company. Reprinted by permission.

each year, along with 3.6 trillion gallons that are released into rivers that flow into the ocean."[51]

Break In Pipe Spews Sewage Near San Diego's Shore

". . .city water officials were forced to continue to pump 170 million to 180 million gallons a day from the Point Loma Wastewater Treatment Plant through the ruptured pipe, which normally carries the treated, but not sanitized, sewage to an outlet 2.5 miles off the coast, where it is carried away by ocean currents."[52]

San Diego Lifts Quarantine On Some Beaches

". . .silt from heavy rains clogged pumps that carried raw sewage from Tijuana, Mexico, to the treatment plant in San Diego. With the pumps clogged, 13 million gallons of raw sewage was carried daily by the Tijuana River into the ocean."[53]

Hot Angelenos Gaze Longingly At Beaches' Forbidden Waves[54]

Lead In Greenland Is Traced To The U.S.

"Lead deposits, which accumulated in soil and snow during the 1960's and 70's, were primarily the result of leaded gasoline emissions originating in the United States. In the 20 years that the Clean Air Act has mandated unleaded

---

[51]   © 1992 by The New York Times Company. Reprinted by permission.

[52]   © 1992 by The New York Times Company. Reprinted by permission.

[53]   © 1992 by The New York Times Company. Reprinted by permission.

[54]   © 1992 by The New York Times Company. Reprinted by permission.

gas used in the United States, the lead accumulation worldwide has diminished significantly. "[55]

GAO Faults Regulators On Reproductive, Developmental Hazards[56]

Could you could eat *anything* from the water below? Supposedly fish caught from the ocean are safer to eat.

Viruses Central To Ocean Life

Teaspoon of Sea Water Contains 1 Billion

By William Booth, Washington Post Staff Writer

Scientists trying to understand the cycles of life and death among the smallest creatures in the world's oceans have just discovered that a single teaspoon of sea water typically contains more than 1 billion viruses- at least 1,000 times, and perhaps 10 million times, more than previously estimated.[57]

---

[55]   © 1993 by The New York Times Company. Reprinted by permission.

[56]   © 1992 by The New York Times Company. Reprinted by permission.

[57]   © 1991 by The Washington Post, Washington, DC. Reprinted with permission. pg. 1

An article from The New York Times reads:

Sewage Bacteria In Food Chain

"Scientists have found evidence that organic material from sewage sludge dumped in the deep sea off New Jersey has entered the food chain of bottom-dwelling animals."[58]

These bottom dwelling animals are eaten by the fish we eat.

Do you think the pregnant women from Michigan mentioned in the following article who ate seafood on a regular basis while pregnant knew their babies would be born with "problems" and "motor deficiencies?" I hope the people who were following who was eating seafood out of Lake Michigan notified people eating the fish of the dangers.

My guess is that the women ate the fish because seafood has been lauded as healthy and they went to the extra trouble to eat fresh seafood because they thought it would be good for their babies.

A hundred years ago, it was. But now, with the state of our polluted environment, which includes the spilling of hundreds of tons of oil, dumping by industries as well as government, accidental spills as well as the dumping of thousands of tons of industrial chemicals and solvents, along with bursting sewers that spew millions of gallons of sewage, fertilizer and pesticide run-off, it has become dangerous to eat seafood.

The practice of dumping tons of sewage into the ocean for 100 years alone puts a tremendous burden on the environment, along with the constant pollution from thousands of antiquated burst sewage pipes spewing sewage into our waterways.

---

[58] Reprinted with permission of The New York Times, New York, NY by Walter Sullivan 11/93.

Fish: A Moving Experience?

A Pennsylvania woman and her son were eating haddock she had "cooked" in their new microwave earlier this year, when they noticed some thin, tan, paper-clip-length worms wiggling around in the uneaten portion.

C. Darrell Lane and colleagues at the Reading Hospital and Medical Center identified the creatures as anisakid worms, which can cause a disease aptly named anisakisasis, resulting in fever, nausea, and abdominal problems.

The worms are usually destroyed by cooking, but microwave owners sometimes undercook their fish. Pacific salmon and Pacific rockfish (red snapper) are most frequently linked to anisakisasis, although other fish from Atlantic and pacific waters also can be infected.

The disease is on the rise in the U.S. which is thought to be attributable to the increased popularity of raw fish dishes like sushi and sashimi.

Experts think that many cases of anisakisasis go unreported, because symptoms are often confused with those of appendicitis.

"Be sure to thoroughly cook your food when you microwave. The fish must be heated through to the core for five minutes at 140 degrees to kill anisakid worms," says Reading's Lane.

J. Amer. Med. Assoc. 260.340, 1988; N.Eng. J. Med. 319:1228. 1988.
© 1988 Nutrition Action Healthletter, published by The Center For Science In the Public Interest, 1875 Connecticut Avenue NW, Suite 300, Washington, DC 20009. Reprinted with permission.

Whether cooked or raw, on your plate or distilled into oil capsules, fish is "hot" these days. Maybe it's a little too hot.

The message to eat more seafood is everywhere; we get it from our doctors, in newspaper articles, on television programs and radio talk shows. In fact, it seems the more we try to cut back on saturated fat in our diets, the more fish we consume.

Does it also mean the more contaminants we put in our bodies?

Good Fish...Bad Fish

FISHING FOR SAFE SEAFOOD

(Continued from page 1)

The health benefits of fish are undeniable. It is an excellent source of protein, B vitamins, and trace minerals. It is also low in saturated fat, yet high in omega-3 fatty acids, which may reduce the risk of heart disease. And in a perfect world that would be just fine.

But there's a problem: Many of the chemicals we introduce into the environment eventually work themselves into lakes, streams, and coastal waters. There, they are ingested by simple forms of marine life and small fish, which in turn are eaten by larger fish. In this way, the chemicals slowly work their way up the food chain. Eventually, they end up in your Blackened Catfish or Trout Almondine.

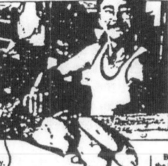

DANGERS OF THE DEEP

How serious is the threat from contaminated fish? Larry Skinner, principal fish and wildlife ecologist with the New York Department of Environmental Conservation, puts it this way: "Your chances of getting cancer from eating a weekly eight-ounce meal of trout caught in Lake Ontario is about the same as your lifetime risk of being murdered in the United States today—about 1 in 200." And if you're eating fish caught in New York's Hudson River, Skinner says the odds are even worse.

Fortunately, commercial fishing of trout from Lake Ontario is banned, and you'd have to be desperately hungry to eat a fish caught in the polluted Hudson. But these are only the most blatant examples. To one degree or another, fish from any body of water are potential repositories of industrial chemicals, pesticides, or toxic metals.

Of course, fish can also be tainted with microorganisms or natural toxins. This biological contamination (usually from raw or spoiled fish or shellfish) accounts for about a quarter of all food poisoning cases reported in the U.S. each year.

THE BAD GUYS

Industrial Chemicals. Among the worst offenders are polychlorinated biphenyls, or PCBs, which have been used for years in lubricants and coolants. Although the manufacturing of PCBs was banned in the United States in 1979, the pollutant continues to show up in high concentrations in wildlife and fish.

In 1984 researchers at Wayne State and other universities examined infants of women who reported regularly eating an average of two or three meals per week of PCB-contaminated fish from Lake Michigan. At birth, the babies showed weak reflexes and sluggish movements, as well as other signs of "worrisome" behavioral development.[1]

And as if that weren't enough: Most of the estimated cancer risk of eating fish also comes from PCB contamination.[2]

Pesticides. In 1963 the Food and Drug Administration found DDT in 334 of the 386 samples of domestic fish it tested, even though the use of this "probable human carcinogen" was halted in 1972.

But Alan Mearns, an ecologist with the National Oceanographic and Atmospheric Administration (NOAA), says that "DDT levels have declined nationwide, and continue to decline."

Another frequently found fish contaminant and probable cancer-causer is chlordane, which has been widely used to control termites. The "probable" label (which PCBs also have been tagged with) means that the substance causes cancer in animals, but that sufficient evidence in humans is still lacking.

But "sufficient evidence" isn't easy to get. "We don't run controlled cancer studies on humans," explains Sherry Sterling, chief of the Health Sciences section of the Office of Waste Programs Enforcement at the EPA. "We rely on animals as a model for the human system."

© 1988 Nutrition Action Healthletter, published by The Center For Science In the Public Interest, 1875 Connecticut Avenue NW, Suite 300, Washington, DC 20009. Reprinted with permission.

People who eat raw fish infected with a worm called *Diphyllobothrium*, can get a rare form of B_{12} deficiency. The tapeworm goes to the human intestine, where it lives and eats all the B_{12} before it gets in the person's system, thus causing the deficiency.

Some other upsetting events:

FDA Warns Of Toxins
In Some Crab Organs

"High levels of domoic acid can cause amnesic shellfish poisoning. The first symptoms are abdominal cramps, diarrhea and nausea. Neurological symptoms, including headaches, dizziness, disorientation, seizures, breathing difficulty and memory loss may occur within 48 hours in severe cases."[59]

Tighten The Rules On Seafood Safety

"Because hundreds of chemicals such as DDT, PCB's and dioxin remain in our waters, seafood is the largest dietary source of toxic chemicals and pesticides. In a 1991 study, the National Academy of Sciences warned that tuna, swordfish and other ocean fish may contain such high levels of mercury that eating them may be a risk for pregnant women and children."[60]

Study Of Retail Fish Markets Finds Wide
Contamination And Mislabeling

"The group found that 34 samples were spoiled, 50 were contaminated with fecal coliforms and 8 of 20 samples of swordfish had more than the permissible level of mercury. PCB's, or polychlorinated biphenyls, which have been found to cause cancer in laboratory animals, contaminated almost

---

[59]   © 1992 by The Washington Post, Washington, DC. Reprinted with permission.

[60]   © 1992 by The New York Times Company. Reprinted by permission.

43 percent of the salmon in the study, half of the whitefish and 25 percent of the swordfish. Mercury, which affects the development of the nervous system, was found in 18 of the swordfish samples. The cleanest fish in terms of PCB's, mercury and pesticides were the sole and flounder."[61]

Chemicals That Taint Seafood

"Last year, retailers and distributors voluntarily stopped selling shark in Minnesota after state officials found levels of methylmercury that exceeded federal guidelines in 24 of the 39 samples that it tested." "What is known is the impact of high levels of methylmercury on human reproduction."[62]

Suppose you were out of town with friends and one of you suggested crabbing and you guys happened to be unlucky enough to be at one of the 2,400 beaches in America that had been closed. Say someone took the sign down to hang on their bedroom wall as a souvenir, and you didn't get to read it? And you went ahead and crabbed and cooked the crabs just five minutes so they could be tender and delicious and succulent?

This happened to me twenty years ago. I crabbed with my friends but I did not eat any, and everyone who ate crabs became violently ill. Fortunately, no one died. I have not eaten a crab comfortably since. Because my family loves seafood and thinks I am overcautious about my health, I often get to sit back and watch various ones of them get sick after eating their seafood dinners.

When I point out that it could be the seafood, they say, naw, it smelled and tasted fresh, so it must have been something else, like the mayonnaise in the potato salad. The truth is, the mayonnaise is far less likely to cause problems than the seafood.

I'm not trying to alarm you, but merely to inform you, because what could happen is you could end up very sick, or dead. So be aware, especially when

---

[61]   © 1992 by The New York Times Company. Reprinted by permission.

[62]   © 1992 by The Washington Post, Washington, DC Healthplus. Reprinted with permission.

eating raw or undercooked seafood. And people you ask about the water in little towns don't always know about such things, so don't put your life in their hands. Eat seafood only from reputable sources.

Another of the ecological devastations from the past few years was:

2,400 Beach Closings Tied To Old Sewers[63]

How would you like to eat some crabs from one of those beaches? Crabs, shrimp and clams live in shallow water, which is usually more polluted. I happen to be familiar with some of the areas mentioned in some of the reports I read about pollution. I know people who go fishing and crabbing in them.

I sent one of them a copy of an article about pollution in the area where he goes crabbing and he called me and said, "Oh, they won't let that go on. The government will clean that up right away." I said, "We have to get off our butts and do our jobs as citizens and protectors of our planet!"

From 1987-1991 there was an abundance of reports of people finding medical wastes on beaches up and down the East and West coasts. Often vials contaminated with AIDS were found, and many times it was reported that they were found by children who got up early on summer mornings to go crabbing. Following are some of them. The next one is from The Washington Post. The headline read:

More Needles Wash Ashore In Arundel

"The wastes, including more than 100 medical syringes with needles attached, condoms and some vials containing blood, were found Wednesday and today on the shore of Rockwood Beach, a residential area southeast of Baltimore.

---

[63]   © 1991 by The New York Times Company. Reprinted by permission.

"The probe was prompted by the discovery of about 400 syringes, some with needles attached, in Baltimore's outer harbor last month.[64]

One state that got on the ball and passed legislation against this kind of dumping was Maryland.

Would you eat seafood from the water mentioned below? How can you be sure that the seafood you eat did not come from this kind of water since there is no regulation guaranteeing its purity? Sounds like Russian roulette to me. Some of the headlines read:

More Needles Wash Ashore In Arundel Contamination[65]

Medical Debris Washes Up in Arundel[66]

Water systems in 35 states were tested and it was discovered that 19 percent of 18,157 systems were tainted with toxic chemicals. Of the toxins found, 190 out of 2,110 were harmful.

By 1988, oil spills were so common they sometimes did not even make the front page headline! I noticed a couple of times when I saw a reference made to the oil spill on the front page, then the page number where the story could be found.

Over and over I have seen sand replaced at beaches at astronomical costs. How did it get contaminated in the first place? What makes anyone think that what contaminated the sand the first time is not going to re-contaminate it? The cleanup needs to be complete, which means the sources of contamination need to be removed and existing contamination needs to be cleaned up. Then the sand

---

[64]   © 1988 by The Washington Post, Washington, DC. Reprinted with permission.

[65]   © 1988 by The Washington Post, Washington, DC. Reprinted with permission.

[66]   © 1990 by The Washington Post, Washington, DC. Reprinted with permission.

needs to be replaced. What do we do with the contaminated sand? Clean it up and recycle it.

CNN reported that there are 439,999 abandoned toxic waste sites in the USA. How do you know that you are not living next door to one? All the health precautions in the world would not save you if you were. National Public Radio reported that your chances of getting cancer are 100 times greater than average if you eat seafood twice a week.

A Government Accounting Office Study in 1987 found that three out of four toxic waste sites are located in African-American and Hispanic communities. Also, three out of five African-Americans and Hispanics live in a community that contains toxic wastes.

In light of new evidence, I say who says it is an absolute that we need to eat seafood? Yes, it was fine to eat seafood as long as it was safe, but now that we know how we have polluted the seafood's home, how can we continue to consume it safely?

Considering that a teaspoon of sea water has possibly 10 million times more viruses than scientists had previously speculated, and considering the fact that viruses are toxic to the human body, it seems obvious that, as we have heavily polluted our waterways for the last hundred years, dumping tons and tons of junk into our waters, that seafood may no longer be good for human consumption unless it is farm grown or from an unpolluted area. And where is there one?

And unless you stood there and watched what went into the water for the last 100 years, no one really knows what went into it. Worse, reported cases are only a fraction of actual cases of pollution!

The problem with our world pollution has been that if we were not there when the million gallons of oil were dumped into the ocean, we were less affected than the people who witnessed it first hand. However, national news coverage brings disasters into our living rooms so we feel the devastations more. But soon, except for a few oil stains on crabs or shrimp, we forget the spill and hope it never happens again.

Nor did we hear about the many, many like incidents that occurred all over the world for a hundred years when there was no national news coverage. Once it happens, the pollution is there, but almost invisible. We are so busy living our own lives, with not enough time in the day as it is, we forget about it. Our children won't. I don't know if they will be able to forgive us.

The incidents included here are only a small sampling of some of the catastrophes that have led our planet to its present polluted state. Multiply these instances times the countries polluting, times one hundred years, and it begins to become apparent that we must clean up the messes we have made.

CDC: Public Pools Fail 4 out of 5 Safety Inspections
Condensed from *NEWSER*, By Evann Gastaldo, Newser Staff, Posted Jan 20, 2011 1:14 PM CST

Watch Out: That Dog, Cat, Rabbit, in Your Bed Could Kill You
You might even get the plague from your furry friends
 Curling up with your dog or cat at the end of a tough day might not feel so warm and fuzzy after reading this: Allowing your pets to sleep in your bed could actually kill you, according to veterinary scientists. A new study shows that those who sleep with their dogs and cats have a higher chance of contracting parasites or any number of illnesses—including the plague, Aol News reports. Also a no-no, if you want to play it safe: kissing your pets or letting them lick you.
Some disturbing examples: a 9-year-old who got the plague from his cat, a couple who got multiple staph infections from their dog, a woman who got meningitis from kissing her pet's face, and two people who died after their pets, a cat and dog respectively, licked their open wounds.

A word to grass cutters, beauticians, aesthetitians, massage therapists, health practitioners, food handlers, nursery workers, construction workers, and those who touch others or inhale things in their work: *You need to wear gloves and a mask.* Everything you inhale goes into your brain immediately. If you don't wear protective gear, such as a mask, then you may be inhaling some things that will stay with you permanently and eventually kill you. So be aware, protect yourself. Use gloves when touching patients or raw vegetation, both loaded with microbes that will start to grow in you. Touching 1,000 patients gives you microbes from 1,000 individuals. We will all live longer healthier lives if we follow this rule.

TAP WATER

Usually, the water that runs through household faucets comes from rainwater, and water that has run off from rivers, lakes and streams. Unfortunately, in addition to the sewage we dump into our waterways, antiquated and bursting sewage pipes leak millions more gallons into our waterways. In addition, millions of gallons of petrochemical spills, lead from cars, pesticides, fertilizer runoff, illegal dumping, pollution from factories and industries, leaking tank farms, coliforms from humans and animals and fallout from nuclear tests and nuclear power plants all can contaminate our water supply as well. All the cities along the Mississippi dump their sewage into it. California and Mexico also have been dumping millions of gallons of raw slightly-treated sewage into the ocean for decades, and continue to do so. Then there are the chemicals used to purify our drinking water, which include chlorine, fluorine, lime, alum, **sodium aluminates and other toxins.** In addition, tap water often contains **toxic substances like asbestos, cyanides, arsenic, lead, mercury, cadmium** That means that structured mineral water or water that is 7.2-6 pH should be consumed or ¼ teasp of Himalayan sea salt added. Here is a good structured water maker: http://www.swaterunit.com/

Sodium fluoride is extremely toxic to the human body. It is about 1,000 times more toxic than sodium chloride, or what we know as table salt. Sodium fluoride is added to our drinking water to prevent tooth decay in the masses.

Adding fluoride to anything makes the total explosive, active. It is so active, in fact that it cannot be kept in bottles because it eats through. Just a dab too much causes convulsions, comma or death!

According to studies the minimum safe dose is one milligram per day. It has been proved over and over that women who get more than 2 mg. of fluorine per day are more prone to bear defective children. So why is this substance in our drinking water? It is much safer and healthier to use hydrogen peroxide and ozone, two natural, safe substances to clean our water and protect our teeth.

Root canals are a primary cause of chronic disease

https://www.naturalhealth365.com/**root_canals**.html

What is a **root canal** treatment and could this be the cause of chronic disease? ... the pro-oxidant toxins of **root canals** ... mercury is an extremely **DEADLY** ...

Root Canals are deadly? - Dental Health Message Board ...

https://**www.healthboards.com**/.../201098-**root-canals-deadly**.html

Aug 22, 2004 · Hi. Just read about one of the head guys who pioneered the **root canal**process, now saying it's not safe. I had to cut this down quite a bit cause they

The Dangerous Truth About Root Canals | ...

undergroundhealthreporter.com › Breaking News

What Are The Dangers of A **Root Canal**? You may have a colony of bacteria in your mouth that you aren't even aware of, especially if you haven't heard about

Are Root Canals Dangerous? - Scott Taylor DDS

www.puresimpledental.com/**root-canals**-alternatives

Are **Root Canals** Dangerous? ... **Root Canals** Can Lead to Heart, ... this ligament can serve as a breeding ground for **deadly** bacteria.

- **http://www.curetoothdecay.com/Dentistry/dentist_hal_huggins.htm**
- **Dental Implants Deadly:**
- Allergy related to dental implant and its clinical significance

https://www.ncbi.nlm.nih.gov/pmc/articles/PMC3753052/Proxy Highlight

Aug 19, 2013 ... Keywords: dental implant, allergy, titanium, corrosion ... as swelling, may involve the upper respiratory tract, and be dangerous for the patient.

Dental implants can cause nerve damage, warns study - BBC News

www.bbc.com/news/health-18366437Proxy Highlight

Jun 8, 2012 ... Dentists are not being vigilant when carrying out implant surgery and are failing to inform patients about the risks of nerve damage, a study in ...

1.A Tooth Infection Can Be Deadly

https://drnemeth.com/a-tooth-infection-can-be-deadly/Proxy Highlight

Feb 8, 2017 ... TOOTH INFECTION. Most of us have had a toothache at one time or another and our first inclination is to wait and see if it eases. or goes away.

2.Fatal air embolism during dental implant surgery: a report of three ...

https://www.ncbi.nlm.nih.gov/pubmed/2295094Proxy Highlight

Fatal air embolism during dental implant surgery: a report of three cases. ... 1987, 11 patients underwent insertion of mandibular dental prostheses by the same

You can copy and paste links into your browser if they don't work..

Chapter 17

> # *WHAT WE CAN DO TO PROTECT OURSELVES*

There are a number of things that can be done to rid the body of the toxins that we have been unknowingly polluting it with. They can build up, in some cases, like an overdose of petrochemicals, and eventually destroy it the same way a buildup of tars from cigarette smoking destroys the lungs, and subsequently, the person. *The effects from a petrochemical overdose become evident a lot faster.*

Aerobic exercises, dance, meditation, Yoga, massage, homeopathic medicines, eating garlic and taking oxygen and eating oxygen-rich foods (fruits and vegetables) are all recommended for strengthening the immune system in order for the body to function at optimum levels. Recently it has been confirmed that taking trace elements like vitamins and minerals protect the body greatly from chronic diseases and illnesses, and that some vitamin and mineral deficiencies can cause serious health problems.

In order to strengthen the immune system, we need to fully activate it on a regular basis. When the activities above are done for a sustained amount of time, usually twenty minutes is the minimum, the immune system becomes fully activated. Stimulating the immune system in this way has become recognized as the fountain of youth because of the other benefits associated with it like raising heart rate, moving lymph fluids, oxygenating the blood, aiding metabolism, lowering blood pressure, eliminating depression and many others. Check with your doctor before starting any exercise program.

Exercise without massage is not recommended. No matter how gradually you start, you are going to end up with some spots on your body that need kinks worked out. Muscle waste products can cause pain and discomfort. Massage is especially essential for weight-lifters. A sprain or injury can be healed in a matter of weeks or days using massage to heal it.

Having a massage triggers a switch much like the switch on a light and turns on the immune system. Then a number of things happen, the body becomes fully oxygenated causing the brain to make endorphins, the pleasure hormones that heal and fill us with a sense of peace and ecstasy. Then the sweeping housecleaning process commences and, with the massage as a catalyst, our body heals itself and the increased flow of lymph fluid and killer cells dissolves toxins, moves putrefying fluids, mucous and congestion and imparts a natural high from the relief of tension and pent-up energy.

You have learned in the previous chapters that we are exposed to unavoidable environmental hazards in our lives everyday ranging from pesticides, PCB's, toxic chemicals like lead, mercury and cadmium, cigarette smoke, people with deadly debilitating contagious diseases like drug-resistant TB, AIDS, hepatitis-B and typhoid. It is comforting to know that there are things like massage that we can get to help strengthen our immune systems and help our bodies fight back by destroying toxins, healing, revitalizing and easing tension and fatigue.

In fact you can make yourself into a *super-immune* individual. One of the most important aspects of achieving this is your mental attitude towards yourself. I don't just look like I'm 20, I feel like it! How I feel about it is very important. If you like yourself, are optimistic, conscientious, can forgive yourself for past mistakes and can use your mind to envision your body stronger, your chances for surviving and living a higher quality of life increase greatly.

> *Our Soils Have Been Declared*
> *Depleted Of The Vitamins And*
> *Minerals Needed For Good*
> *Health Since 1937*

According to a **1937** report from the Department of Health and Human Services, our soil was so depleted then of the essential minerals necessary for the foods we eat to give us what we need to maintain minimum health that we would have had to eat ten times more than we normally ate to get the essential vitamins and minerals we needed from it.

How much more depleted do you think our soils have become since 1937? The fact that this minor tidbit of information is obscured kills thousands of people every year. For if those mothers and fathers knew what the deficiency in our food was doing to their health and their children's, it would be corrected in a flash. Certainly modern agriculture, which has the capacity to enrich the soil, use crop rotation, kelp and natural fertilizers can produce healthy food, but have you seen any of these labels on food?

Most modern chronic diseases can be traced to deficiency. Even minor deficiencies of vitamins and minerals can cause severe illness. We only have to look back at history when deficiency diseases like beri (a B-vitamin deficiency disease), and pellagra (a niacin-deficiency disease) were killing thousands to see the effect of deficiencies. Not much has changed, since people who live predominately on processed foods are still chronically undernourished, usually obese, and suffering and dying needlessly.

For the first time in history, the ultra-conservative **Journal of The American Medical Association** has published a paper that recommends "vitamin supplements" as a way of **preventing** atherosclerosis and heart disease (JAMA, Aug. 19, 1992-pgs. 877-881.) This follows a widely publicized study reported in the May 1992 issue of the journal **Epidemiology** that showed that supplemental vitamin C could increase average life span in men by six years.

© 1993 by Life Extension Foundation, Box 229120, Hollywood, FL. Reprinted with permission

---

I have been taking vitamin C for more than fifteen years and the only time I begin to get a cold is when I miss my vitamin C for more than two days. It also seems to keep other ills away.

Researchers have proved that people who live on hamburgers, french fries, pizza, high-fat, **salty,** sugary foods don't live as long as people who eat mostly fruits, vegetables, **nuts**   If your diet consists of a lot of bacon and eggs, fries, fried chicken or fried foods, sodas and burgers, you are headed for the crash landing.

Some recent headlines in The New York Times report:

CHEMISTS LEARN WHY VEGETABLES ARE GOOD FOR YOU

Certain Plant Ingredients Can Inhibit Cancers[67]

CHEMISTS LEARN WHY VEGETABLES IN DIET HELP PEOPLE AVOID CANCER[68]

VITAMINS WIN SUPPORT AS POTENT AGENTS OF HEALTH

Focus On Deficiency Diseases Widens To Cholesterol, Cancer and Chronic Disorders.[69]

AFTER YEARS OF SKEPTICISM, VITAMINS WIN SUPPORT AS AGENTS OF HEALTH

Discovering How Diet Aids Health.[70]

Newly Suspected Benefits of Vitamins In The Body

---

[67] © 1993 by The New York Times Company. Reprinted by permission.

[68] © 1990 by The New York Times Company. Reprinted by permission.

[69] © 1991 by The New York Times Company. Reprinted by permission.

[70] © 1991 by The New York Times Company. Reprinted by permission.

Vitamins, essential chemicals found in food and sometimes made in the body, may have roles beyond preventing deficiency diseases.[71]

SHARP CUT IN SERIOUS BIRTH DEFECT IS TIED TO VITAMINS IN PREGNANCY
Survey of 23,000 Women Is Termed A Landmark.[72]

VITAMIN C LINKED TO HEART BENEFIT
It May Also Help Prevent An Early Death From Other Diseases, Study Says.[73]   Stick with Liposomal vitamin C for best results.

VITAMIN PACK IS FOUND TO AID ELDERLY
Immune System Improved.[74]

Go for vitamins made from whole foods and fermented for best results.

Nutritionists Look At Supplements As Weapons Against Chronic Illness[75]

When you consume overly processed foods you get less of the essential nutrients that your body so desperately needs, so your body will continue to crave food, trying to fill the void. This leads to obesity and bad health, which could be

---

[71]   © 1992 by The New York Times Company. Reprinted by permission.

[72]   © 1989 by The New York Times Company. Reprinted by permission.

[73]   © 1992 by The New York Times Company. Reprinted by permission.

[74]   © 1992 by The New York Times Company. Reprinted by permission.

[75]   © 1993 by The Washington Post, Washington, DC. Reprinted with permission

avoided if pure, whole fresh foods were consumed as nature intended. If you must eat cakes, pies, muffins, make them with coconut or almond flour.

Since our food is incapable of filling all of our body's requirements for nourishment we have to go the extra distance and be responsible for making sure our bodies get it's needed requirements. A good way to help that is by juicing veggies and fruits.

If we all wised up and stopped buying junk food, manufacturers would stop making them. The only reason they are out there is because there is a demand for them. Many food manufacturers don't know that fruits and veggies are not to be mixed together in order for proper digestion to occur.

Cayenne Pepper Is The "King Of All Herbs"

Stop Serious Bleeding in 10 Seconds – *Keep This Herb in Your First Aid Kit*

*I*t does not matter if the wound is external or internal, an individual can internally drink a cup of warm tea with a few shakes of cayenne pepper stirred into it or externally apply cayenne powder onto the wound. The bleeding will generally stop after 10 seconds. It appears that from the top of the head to the bottom of the feet, cayenne pepper equalizes the blood pressure to keep the pressure from the hemorrhage area, allowing the wound to clot naturally. **CAUTION**: *Some individuals are extremely sensitive to cayenne. Too much can be fatal.* If you are a first time user, start with very small amounts, like 1/8 teasp to an 8oz cup of soup. To still get the benefits and neutralize the choke factor, add 1 teaspoon of apple cider vinegar to the cup. Gradually increase your dosage for additional benefits. Most of those I have seen who are sensitive to eating cayenne are able to take it in pill form.

Pepper. It is more powerful than any other with hundreds of benefits.

The red pepper has been used for thousands of years for healing and has produced tremendous results treating baffling symptoms. Cayenne has been used to help relieve migraines, reduce cholesterol, alleviate asthma symptoms, fight infections, stop a heart attack, indigestion, and much more.

Every child's birthright should be that he has proper nutrition; his brain cannot grow and function properly without it. Every child needs to be taught the golden rule and afforded every educational opportunity. This world would be far more perfect if people were not allowed to drop-out but forced to finish their education. We have a whole underclass of uneducated people in this country causing havoc in our cities and on our streets and making it unsafe for everyone.

Many of these people prefer to rob and steal rather than work for 4 dollars an hour. Educational rehabilitation should be mandatory for prisoners instead of spending 60,000 dollars a year to house a criminal. Indeed, it is discriminatory to teach prisoners skills like auto mechanics and construction. If we fed their minds and gave them two years of psychology and philosophy, these things can drive the criminal out of a person.

A child's parents should have a responsibility to him, and to themselves, to know what proper nutrition is and its importance and the value of becoming a productive and respected member of society. This is basic survival. And look how the species that has not digested this information survives. They die needlessly of cancers, diabetes, strokes, heart attacks that should never happen.

Organic...

By Karen Nelson Baker

Aren't "organic foods" just another yuppie fad? Why should I bother?

In today's health-conscious world, it seems anyone can make the headlines by claiming to discover a new "miracle food." But organically grown food is not just another fad. It is a vital change in the way that Americans grow and consume food.

Organic food is purer and safer than food that has been sprayed with chemical fertilizers and pesticides. Organic agriculture also addresses a host of sustainability issues and environmental concerns, such as loss of farmland productivity and depletion of fossil resources.

Do my purchasing habits really make a difference?

Yes! When you buy organic, you support the market for organic agriculture. You allow organic farmers to make a living, and encourage non-organic farmers to make the switch.

A 1988 Harris Poll showed that 85% of people in the United States said they would buy organic food if it cost the same as non-organic, and half would even pay more. If all of these Americans lived up to their words by demanding and buying organic food, chemical agriculture would be all but banished from contaminating our country.

Shopping (and eating) organic means that we are taking responsibility for our

part in the American food production system. It is every bit as important as supporting other good works with our time, energy, or money.

Isn't organic agriculture still new and experimental?

Some organic growing techniques are indeed new, but many more represent a return to "tried and true." The

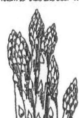

current American food production system, so heavily dependent on petroleum based fertilizers and toxic pesticides, only began to dominate American agriculture after World War II. Many strategies now being rediscovered, such as crop rotation and manure spreading, were basic to farm practice not very long ago.

How are organic foods more healthy?

Pesticide residues cause 50,000 cases of pesticide poisoning each year. Exposure to pesticide residues can cause cancer, birth defects, and damage to many body organs. They are dangerous to consumers and even more so to the workers and farmers who must apply them.

Organically grown foods contain no toxic chemicals, because they were grown without the use of pesticides, on a farm where agrichemicals have not been used for three or more years.

How are organic foods better for the environment?

The Living Soil

Soil is not just dirt. Healthy soil is a complex and fragile community of live microorganisms. In fact, just one teaspoonful of good garden soil has a microorganism population larger than the earth's human population. A healthy soil community provides nutrients for crops and protects them against disease, erosion, and drought.

76   ORGANIC OR WHAT? is reprinted with permission of The Bethesda Co-op News, the free newspaper of the Bethesda Co-op since 1975. Located at 6500 Seven Locks Road, Cabin John, Maryland 20818. Phone (301) 320-2530.

Or What?

Under typical commercial agriculture, however, harsh Nitrogen-Potassium-Phosphorus (NPK) fertilizers are used, which eventually kill off the naturally occurring soil life. A vicious cycle is established, in which ever more fertilizer is required for ever more depleted soil. By losing its microorganisms, the soil becomes more tightly packed, encouraging fertilizer runoff and topsoil erosion. Finally, since fertilizers are based on petroleum, they are expensive for the farmer, and they contribute to our national oil addiction.

Not All Fertilizers Are Created Equal

Of course, organic farmers also need to nourish the soil. But rather than harsh petroleum-based chemicals, they use compost and green manure. Composts are organically recycled plant

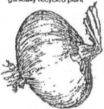

wastes that are also rich in microorganisms. Green manures are crops that are plowed back into the soil to enrich it. Legumes are especially important as green manures since they "fix" atmospheric nitrogen into a form that is usable to plant crops.

Weeds and Pests

American agribusiness gets rid of weeds, insects, and other pests by poisoning them — and often us as well. These chemicals are dangerous to the farmers and workers who apply them; they contaminate our soil and groundwater; they can be concentrated in the food chain, resulting in damage to wildlife and contamination of milk and dairy products; and they linger on in residues that are dangerous to consumers.

Organic farmers know that they have a battery of other options. Cover crops and mulches are used to smother weeds before they can get a good start. Soil solarization destroys weed seed by heating the soil under plastic. Crop rotation helps to break up the life cycles of pests. Predator insects, such as lady bugs, praying mantises, and predator wasps, can also be encouraged to return, or purchased for release on the farm.

So Why Don't More Farmers Do It?

Although the number of organic farmers tripled between 1988 and 1990, they

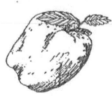

still account for less than three percent of all farmers in the United States. A number of barriers obstruct the adoption of organic farming practices, including:

* Federal crop subsidies — support payments to farmers — to a large extent determine both the crops and the methods of U.S. farmers, and they subsidize the status quo. The subsidies are based on planting a single crop per field. Cover cropping and crop rotation are not encouraged, and in some cases not even allowed. There are no government incentives to farm organically.
* Loan agencies and banks, upon which many farmers depend for annual production loans, rarely lend for the "non-traditional" supplies needed by organic

farmers — compost, cover crop seed, or new cultivation equipment, for example.
* There is little information or advice for organic farmers. University research, often funded by agrichemical businesses, focuses primarily on chemical-intensive farming. Similarly, only one-half of one percent of the U.S. Department of Agriculture research and education budget is devoted to non-chemical or sustainable farming methods.
* Agrichemical businesses themselves are very powerful. Control in these industries is extremely concentrated. For example, between 1972 and 1982, the top four pesticide manufacturers increased their market share from 33 to 59 percent.

How Do I Know Organic Food Really Is?

Several types of labelling exist to verify the claim of organically grown food. Certified Organically Grown means that the food is grown in accordance with strict standards, and independently verified by on-farm inspections, soil and water testing, and careful record-keeping. Generally, Certified Organic farmland must be free from agrichemical use for at least three years. This label guarantees that the best available, ecologically sound methods were used to grow the crop and to enhance soil and other natural resources.

Organically Grown In Accordance with California Health and Safety Code Section 26569.11 refers to the California Organic Food Act of 1979. Food must be grown and processed without synthetic fertilizers or pesticides. The California code is less strict than Certified Organically Grown, since there is no requirement for independent verification (although there is a penalty for misrepresentation).

Transition or Transitional Organic labels identify foods grown in a transition period between chemical and organic agriculture. Since most certifying organizations require a three year wait before a farm will be certified, buying transitional organic foods will help support farmers who are trying to change. Many transitional farmers do use organic sprays while they are building soil fertility. These include

fertilizing sprays from kelp or compost, soap sprays to control pests, and oil or mineral sprays to suffocate disease spores and pest eggs. Unlike many agrichemicals, these sprays are not systemic — that is, they are not taken up by the roots and incorporated into plant tissues. They break down easily in the presence of oxygen, air and microorganisms, avoiding lingering residues in food or the environment.

Some food labels, however, should be viewed with caution: unsprayed (although

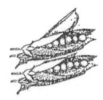

the crop was not sprayed, pesticides may have been applied to the seeds or through irrigation water, and herbicides and fertilizers may also have been used); pesticide-free (the farmer's or agribusiness' claim that no pesticides were used); and Integrated Pest Management or IPM (ideally, IPM farmers use synthetic pesticides only as a last resort).

Sources:

"American Farming: Changes and Questions," in The Washington Spectator, Vol 16, No. 17 (Sept 15, 1990), pp. 1-3.

"Growing Concerns: Questions and Answers about Organic Farming," from Organic Food Matters, Committee for Sustainable Agriculture, pp. 7 - 11.

Francis Moore Lappe, Diet for a Small Planet, 10th Anniversary Edition, Ballantine, 1982.

Jon Naar, Design for a Livable Planet, Harper and Row, 1990.

Karen Nelson Baker is a member of Bethesda Co-op's Recycling Team.

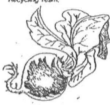

No amount of exercise, fresh foods or proper diet can help you if your body is missing the essential micro-nutrients found in a multi-vitamin and mineral pill. And since it is impossible for our diets to provide them, the only alternative we have is supplements.

In May of 1993 the government of Cuba reported 34,000 cases of mysterious blindness. This phenomenon had started occurring 18 months prior. A team of experts from America were called in. They discovered widespread malnutrition and a toxic substance found in homemade run were to blame.

> ## There Are Lots Of Things
> ## You Can Do

Some things that will greatly increase your ability to fight off disease are: eating the bulk of your diet as whole foods like fruits, veggies, freshly extracted juices and small amounts of protein. Food as medicine will keep you healthy. Organic fresh unadulterated foods contain essential micronutrients that are powerful weapons for health.

Humans have known for 5,000 years about the curative properties of foods. Eating from the four food groups above can keep you healthy and disease-free and increase your life span and its quality. Everywhere you look now there are proclamations from researchers on how certain ingredients in fruits and vegetables and vitamins and minerals help fight cancer and chronic diseases. With proper use of diet, exercise and vitamin and mineral supplements, many chronic illnesses can be prevented.

Genistein is a substance found in people who eat a large amount of vegetables. What it does is prevent the growth of new blood vessels, which tumors need when they are forming. This event effectively prevents them from ever developing. Shark cartilage is used in cancer patients in much the same way. It is recommended that healthy people do not take shark cartilage.

Antioxidants and enzymes found in fruits and vegetables virtually eat up harmful substances like a pac-man game. Broccoli, cabbage, brussels sprouts and cauliflower contain indoles which massively protect us from breast and other cancers. These vegetables also cause the body to make helpful enzymes which prevent cancer from being able to establish itself. Vitamin K, found in broccoli, cabbage and brussels sprouts helps cause blood clotting when we get injured. It also helps prevent the rapid loss of calcium often found in postmenopausal women.

Vitamins, minerals and enzymes are so essential to life that even minor deficiencies can cause serious illness. They keep us healthy by aiding metabolism and the essential biological cellular processes of our bodies. They not only increase the body's ability to fight off disease, they reduce the effects of aging and the incidence of chronic diseases. Researchers are now estimating that man could live to 150-200 years and still be productive. I like that idea about immortality. Let's not rule it out.

Some vitamins are water-soluble and some oil-soluble. Water-soluble vitamins must be taken daily as they are depleted within 72 hours. They are vitamins C and B-complex. Oil-soluble vitamins are A, D, E and K. They are stored in the body from one to four days and can be toxic if taken in improperly high dosages. As a rule, a vitamin and mineral pill will have balanced dosages. Vitamins and minerals are essential for the proper functioning of our bodies. A deficiency of two simple minerals like chromium and magnesium can cause a heart attack. A study found that most heart-attack patients had a chromium and/or magnesium deficiency. Bananas have also been found to help prevent heart attacks.

Magnesium is essential to health and is important in the very essential enzyme systems of the body. A deficiency can cause: disorientation, poor memory, depression, anxiety, whole-body tension, muscle tension, kidney stones, osteoporosis, sudden death after myocardial infarction, rapid heart beat, anorexia, negativism, violent behavior, failure to heal, growth problems, tooth loss, hallucinations, tremors, charley horses, convulsions and a feeling of being ill. In some cases it completely eliminated PMS.

Muscles cannot properly relax if there is a deficiency of magnesium. In addition, it is essential in order for the entire body to fully relax. Many people develop soreness in their necks, backs and legs that can be relieved by taking magnesium. People who were given magnesium after bypass surgery had reduced heart rhythm problems by 50 percent. They also recovered quicker. People who received magnesium after a heart attack had a better chance of surviving. Take it before bed as it acts as a tranquilizer. Take it before a heart attach and the heart attack might not occur. Chromium, potassium and magnesium also help prevent heart attacks.

Naturally alkalizing foods such as vegetables and can help maintain the pH balance in your body, and help you feel healthier overall. And whereas both fruits and veggies have alkalizing properties - vegetables win. Juiced veggies are the top alkali-forming foods that provide massive amounts of essential enzymes, vitamins and minerals

There are too many advantages to taking vitamins and minerals to mention them all here. I have used myself as a guinea pig and I can swear that without my vitamins, I feel like a dishrag no matter how well I eat. Vitamin A, essential for healthy skin and hair, increases resistance to infection and prevents cancer in the organs. Vitamin A, Yohimbine and L-Arginine have been used in separate tests to successfully treat impotence. Some other infection-fighting vitamins are vitamins C and B-complex. Zinc, Goldenseal, Thyme, Capsicum, Echinacea and Comfrey also help fight infection.

Vitamin E has been known to dissolve clots in veins and prevent them from forming. It helps heal and eliminate scar tissue. It helps prevent pulmonary embolism and decreases the body's need for oxygen. It helps circulation and restores capillary permeability to normal. It helps athletes perform better. It is important in that it helps prevent heart attacks and damage from environmental pollution.

If you eat a lot of saturated fats, you need to take vitamin E. Vitamins E, A, D and K are not water soluble, so you could overdose on them. Large amounts of vitamin E raise blood pressure slightly, but the beneficial effects more than set off this risk. To avoid it take between 1-400 IU per day, a safe dose. Vitamins C and B are water soluble and need to be taken everyday.

Taking 100 mg. of vitamin E a day reduces the risk of heart attack by 40 percent. Higher doses boost the immune system and healing and stimulate killer white blood cells. It prevents soreness after a workout and helps prevent bruising.

Folic acid, found in leafy green vegetables and liver, prevents birth defects. It strengthens chromosomes so they can prevent viruses from going deep into the cells and becoming tumors. It is important that women get sufficient amounts of it during the first six weeks of pregnancy.

Women who had deficiencies of folic acid delivered babies with neural-tube defects such as anencephaly, open spine and spina bifida, all ugly conditions. Vitamin D prevents breast, colon and prostrate cancer. Vitamin D is good for depression, bones, skin, breast, ovaries, parathyroid gland, fertility and the pancreas.

Vitamin C is excellent for controlling bacterial as well as viral infections. It helps our cells make interferon and lowers cholesterol about 12 percent after a year of faithful use. It is an antioxidant and required for cellular growth and repair and proper functioning of the adrenal glands. Liposomal C is preferred.

It can cure an infection if given every hour for several hours. It protects against heart disease and reduces the harmful effects of fatty acids and helps the body make the mortar of healthy cells, and therefore reduces cholesterol, since cholesterol only attaches to damaged cells. It has been proved to prevent cancer, prevent and cure infections and stimulate immunity.

It helps wounds to heal and reduces the effects of stress. It along with vitamin A are considered the skin vitamins since vitamin C promotes healthy skin and gums and promotes collagen production and vitamin A aids cellular functions. Vitamin C helps the liver produce P-450, the enzyme that helps convert cholesterol to bile. It works synergistically with vitamin E. Of all the forms of vitamin C available, Liposomal vitamin C is used most efficiently by the body. You also need less of it than normal vitamin C. Other supplements known to be good for skin are amino acids, primrose oil, vitamin B-complex, vitamin E and zinc. Oxygen is very important for healthy skin also.

Selenium deficiency leads to heart attacks, muscular dystrophy and cystic fibrosis. Selenium is an antioxidant that stimulates the immune system and protects our cell's membranes. Only small doses are needed. Overdoses can be toxic.

Deficiencies of the trace elements Lanthanum, Praseodymium, Samarium and Thulium lead to a shortened life span. Sufficient amounts extend life.

Zinc deficiency can lead to birth defects, infertility and chronic infections.

Boron deficiency leads to osteoporosis and arthritis.

Lithium, a trace element, reduces aggressiveness, violence and self-destruction. Lack of it leads to depression, mania, suicidal tendencies, spouse and offspring abuse. The amino acid L-tyrosine converts to norepinephrine in the brain. This chemical produces positive moods and gives motivation and drive and a feeling of well-being. Large doses of B-complex (2-400 mg/day) along with small amounts of amino acids produce a feeling of bliss, a natural high and enhance color perception.

Violent, out of control children were given vitamin and mineral supplements and a proper diet and put into a pink environment (pink calms), and they began to act normal again. Any parent would be grieved to think his kid misbehaved or was unable to learn in school because he did not provide that kid proper nutrition, which includes supplements.

Children who were malnourished had more difficulty learning and paying attention than children who were not. Children who received vitamin supplements had higher IQ's than children who did not. Imagine what these simple facts, if applied in our schools, could do for our school-age children, the men and women of tomorrow.

Whenever I need to stay up late, I take an extra dose of amino acids. They are proteins that are essential to life and permeate   every cell and organ of every living animal. They help protein to work by participating in all the many vital chemical processes of the body. They enable the central nervous system to function properly.

People who take amino acids see the world differently from people who don't. To them, colors are more vibrant and brilliant. Vitamins and minerals are useless without amino acids for they cannot be absorbed and assimilated. Do not take in high dosages. Too much protein can overburden the kidneys and cause problems.

Organic Germanium is a trace element used to treat cholesterol, candidiasis, viral infections, cancer, AIDS and arthritis. It oxygenates tissues. Sources for it are garlic, shiitake mushrooms, onions, ginseng and aloe vera. Use it to promote overall health. Do not take any form of Germanium except organic. An excellent abundant source for it is the herb, garlic, when eaten raw.

It only makes sense that high levels of bad fats in the diet lead to high levels of bad fats in our bloodstreams. This can cause atherosclerosis (blood vessel walls caked with cholesterol and parasites, fats and calcium deposits). Daily apply Rose Beauty cream after a bath or shower has been shown to help reduce this condition.

One of the main reasons for this condition is the typical American fast-food diet, which is loaded with fried food cooked with toxic Canola and vegetable oil, which forms cancer-causing acrylamides. Chronic ingestion of quick sugars causes havoc to our bodies insulin as well as our mental and physical stability.

Essential fatty acids are just that and we need sufficient amounts of them daily. Two tablespoons of olive, avacado, coconut oil daily help prevent heart attacks. Omega-3 foods are believed to help lower the risk for heart disease due to their inflammation-reducing abilities. They also are needed for proper neurological function, cell membrane maintenance, mood regulation and hormone production.

Often it is found when the hair of diabetics is analyzed that the ratio of calcium to zinc is frequently too high. Zinc is a mineral that is needed for insulin activity. Often, high calcium suppresses it. Diabetics are also often found to be low in Manganese.

If quick sugars are eaten in large amounts glycogen is stored (in the liver) or is converted to fatty acids and stored in the body as fat with a little help from your insulin. We know now that the large increase in cardiovascular disease and death is more because of the increased sugar in our diet than any other single factor. To turn off your sugar craving, make sure your get enough chromium in your diet and see if the craving doesn't disappear.

If people eat quick sugars on a regular basis, day after day, the sugar is stored as glycogen or is converted to fats and stored as fats. This process needs insulin. What has been learned is that the large increase in heart disease within the last 100 years is the result of the increased amount of sugar in the American diet.

Sugar not only turns to fat. It also causes adhesiveness of blood platelets. This is the first step in the formation of blood clots and thrombosis. When the blood platelets clump together they become poorly nourished and the blood vessels weaken, allowing cholesterol and fats to invade and narrow the blood vessels further. Exercise and massage would certainly help this condition by oxygenating the cells, blood and blood vessel walls.

The American diet contains too much sugar, fat and salt. It is responsible for the death of more people than ever died on our highways or in our wars. Even young children and teenagers have diabetes   It is not uncommon to hear of teenagers and young adults suffering strokes, when 100 years ago, such a thing was unheard of. This is because of our diets. Any kid who eats burgers and fries three times a day will very likely develop arteriosclerosis, a cholesterol problem, heart disease and a host of other ills.

Kids watch commercials telling them that a candy bar is going to give them energy. So between classes, two hours after lunch they feel hungry and they wolf down two candy bars and drink a can of soda, thinking this is going to give them energy. What this does is give the kid a momentary diabetic shock. He is likely to feel weak, totally wiped out of energy and even a little spacy. If he is healthy, his pancreas will begin functioning normally again and then he will feel hungry as heck!

A wiser snack is four or five pieces of fruit. Don't try to satisfy your hunger with one or two pieces. But five or six pieces will satisfy even the largest appetite for a few hours.

Americans started consuming more saturated fats around the 1900's. Since then, the incidence of heart attacks has tripled. For example, the death rate from heart disease in 1909 was 153 per 100,000. In 1960 that number had nearly tripled to 360 per 100,000.

This is the same time that margarine became a hit with Americans, and its decline is only now occurring since people became aware of the big margarine scam. Liquid polyunsaturated oil, or margarine, is fine as margarine, but when they harden (by hydrogenating it) and put it in sticks, it becomes a saturated fat. So what started out healthy becomes unhealthy. If you need the butter flavor, mix olive oil and butter flavored salt for a safe taste of butter.

Some of the worst oils you can put in your body are re-used oils, rancid oils, saturated fats. hydrogenated fats (like from sticks of margarine) hydrogenated shortenings,

Bad fats in the diet cut down on blood flow and cause the red blood cells to stick together. This reduces the supply of oxygen to the tissues. When the blood becomes weakened in this way, fats and cholesterol invade the damaged cells and shortenings, lard and most animal fats narrow them even more. This is the beginning of clot formation and other degenerative processes.

Here's a funny story that you may not have heard the end of. Many years ago the American Heart Association formally announced that eggs in the American diet were the cause of high cholesterol. Everyone started cutting back on eggs.

But researchers continued studying the egg and they discovered that 50-75 percent of the body's cholesterol is made by the body, and eating eggs did not have that much of an effect on a person's cholesterol level. They discovered that the egg is a superior food (as long as it is not contaminated with viruses or bacteria), that it contained a wide array of essential nutrients, including one of the highest quality proteins found in any food and that the amino acids in the egg helped clear up skin problems, that the lecithin in the egg helped digestion and emulsification of fats.

Then they discovered that we all need cholesterol, and even if you do not eat enough, your liver makes it. Cholesterol is essential for the proper functioning of the body, the manufacture of hormones and to form the bile acids needed to absorb fats. Cholesterol-lowering drugs actually lead to early death.

Essentially, what this all means is that every man, woman and child needs exercise, whole, unprocessed foods and a daily multi-vitamin and mineral to maintain minimum health. Since our soils have been depleted of many of the essential vitamins and minerals needed for our food to give us everything we need from it since 1937, and since it has been proven that vitamins, minerals and the recommended essential amino acids and enzymes are critical for good health, a good multi-vitamin and mineral supplement is essential.

I prefer the Life Extension Multi-Vitamin and mineral and their herbal mix. No other vitamin and mineral pill can touch this one. The Life Extension Foundation also has available anti-aging nutrients and drugs and directories of alternative practitioners. They can be reached at 1-800-822-5388. Another good multi-vitamin and mineral is KAL's Multi Active (KAL, Inc, PO Box 4023, Woodland Hills, CA 91365-4023) which (3 tablets) contain the protective effect of 4 pounds of fruits and vegetables. They can be found in health food stores.

An inexpensive balanced multiple vitamin and mineral is Ultra Vit-Min. with 72 chelated minerals (the Co-Op brand, made by the same people who make a leading brand, for about half the cost of most others) from the Bethesda Co-Op, at 6500 Seven Locks Road, Cabin John MD 20818. Chelated minerals bind with harmful substances and escort them out of the body.

Essential for every man, woman and child also, are: 1-400 mg. of timed release B-complex, 60-1,000 mg. of vitamin C per day, a good natural source of amino acids (like beans and rice, corn or wheat), or a supplement three times a week. Coenzyme Q_{10} and spirulina are helpful for increased vitality and immune system functioning. If you are one of those people looking for one pill to take, take the Life Extension multi-vitamin and mineral tablets.

Do not cheat on eating well and load up on multi-vitamins thinking you can compensate. Do not take more than the recommended dosage thinking more is better. Take the recommended dosage of the vitamin of your choice, but do not take one with every meal, for example, unless the directions specifically say to do so.

To further enhance health, extra B_{12}, acidophilus, oxygen and Km (available from Matol). Km is a potassium mineral supplement   composed of a good choice of healing herbs. This is a potent tonic and should be taken in small amounts once a day or every other day.

Monitor the effect of taking this botanical on your body and adjust your dosage accordingly. Taking a combination of all of the above will make you see life through rose colored glasses because these added nutrients will put you literally in a constant state of bliss! *Food supplements (vitamins and minerals) should be taken with food* unless the directions specifically tell you to do otherwise.

In instances where vitamin C is recommended, Liposomal vitamin C is superior to others. It has all the benefits without the acidity and it is absorbed instantly into the bloodstream and used more efficiently by the body. You also need less of it. Taking the nutrients above will help maintain maximum health and keep your immune system strong and your body functioning smoothly. I chew a simple Papaya enzyme tablet when I don't have raw food to eat with a meal. Digestive enzymes like papaya also dissolve toxins and aid digestion. Never eat cooked food without raw food or enzymes. That is when you fall asleep after eating.

You can supplement with many healing foods like cooked mushooms (never eat them raw) Shiitake and Reishi are the most healing because they make your body produce interferon and beta glucan. Just let your intuition play a role in helping you decide what the extra supplements you get to increase your health will be? It instinctively knows what you need. Somehow we have repressed this ability, but it can be recalled with some effort.

If you come down with an infection, increase vitamin C consumption up to 500-2,000 mg/day until the infection is over. It can be purchased at drug stores, Homeopathic and Apothecary-type pharmacies and health food stores. One quarter of a teaspoon usually equals 1,000 mg. which you should gradually increase your dosage to. During an illness, before surgery, or if a person smokes, higher doses may be needed. Colloidal or Nano silver should be a goto for any illness.

Pycnogenol is a bioflavonoid that used to be prohibitively expensive but which has gone down in price considerably. It is rapidly absorbed and has antioxidant properties that are 50 times greater than vitamin E and 20 times more than vitamin C. It inhibits the enzymes that lead to histamine formation in the body.

Histamine formation can depress the immune system and cause asthma and allergies. Pronogenol carries vitamin C into the cells and stabilizes oxidized vitamin C. It crosses the blood-brain barrier to protect our central nervous system. It is excellent for the skin for it increases and enhances collagen's elasticity and flexibility. There are more than 105 beneficial effects of it.

Bilberry is a flavonoid extract that strengthens capillary beds and protects brain capillaries against hypertension. It reduces the formation of abnormal blood clots by inhibiting platelet aggregation. It has impressively reduced ischemic strokes by its effects on capillary fragility. It improved night vision in 75 percent of people who took it for the problem.

Chlorella contains the highest natural concentrations of cancer-preventing chlorophyll. It contains lots of nucleic acids RNA and DNA that ensure healthy cell metabolism. It detoxifies the body of heavy metals and pesticides and helps clean out the intestines. It is the most potent anti-mutagenic that has ever been found.

Milk thistle extract is an antioxidant that greatly benefits the liver because it contains 85 percent silymarin. Silymarin protects and enhances liver function because it stimulates liver protein synthesis and prevents factors that cause liver damage.

Ginkgo biloba is one of the hottest mind enhancers used in Europe. It also prevents disease, improves the mind and protects the vascular system. It should be taken for no more than 90 days at a time.

Astragalus increases interferon production and is the most potent immune system enhancing herb. It helps allergies, psoriasis, cancer, Epstein-Barr Syndrome, and acts as an adaptogen to relieve stress-induced immune system suppression. It lengthens telomeres, which extend life.

Ginseng enhances mental, athletic, immune system and sexual functioning. It increases vitality and aids in stress management.

Green tea and green tea extract capsules contain polyphenols which reduce the incidence of cancer, heart disease, stroke, hypertension and infections. It is also used to treat asthma, diabetic cataracts, alcoholic hepatitis and liver diseases and heart disease. It, along with astragalus are two very important immune boosting herbs.

Green tea reduced blood glucose levels and plasma insulin levels in animals who received it along with starch or glucose. It reduces the risk of bacterial infection and helps prevent dental caries. It has a potent effect on common bacterias. It is prescribed by oriental doctors to treat viruses, colds and flu. Studies showed that it greatly inhibited the influenza virus.

Our brains are composed of 30 percent Lecithin. It metabolizes fat and prevents cholesterol from collecting on artery walls.

Down through the ages, crying has been regarded as a source of purification and detoxification. Primitive people knew this long before scientists analyzed tears and found that they always contain an abundance of toxins. Where do these toxins come from? They accumulate in our bodies from the toxins we breathe in from our polluted air. They accumulate in the side of the neck and nasal passages. To eliminate them, watch a good tear-jerker (a good tear-jerker differs from a tear-jerker in that it elicits lots of tears), everyone has their favorite, and notice how much emotional relief and alleviation of shoulder and neck stiffness and pain you experience.

Chapter 18

HEAL THE BODY
NATURALLY WITH
HOMEOPATHY

Homeopathy is an ancient natural healing system. References to it have been found in writings as far back as 500 bc. It offers an alternative to drugs by using specially prepared microdoses of some natural substance, usually an herb, root or mineral to stimulate the body's own natural immune response. It is a sophisticated method of individualizing small doses in order to initiate our body's healing response. Homeopaths believe that body and mind are inseparable.

The beauty of homeopathic medicine is that it is absolutely safe, and self-treatment is possible with a little research. Two good books on the subject are **Discovering Homeopathy,** published by North Atlantic Books, Berkeley CA., 1991 by Dana Ullman, and **Homeopathic Medicine At Home** by M. Panos.

It is very important to remember that homeopathic treatments should be determined according to the symptoms that the body is presenting. Even though some remedies are universally used to treat certain ailments, the totality of symptoms should be considered when prescribing treatment.

> Besides offering effective treatment for infectious diseases, homeopaths provided care for a wide range of acute and chronic disease. The observation that patients under homeopathic care lived longer than others led some life insurance companies to offer a 10 percent discount to homeopathic patients.[77] There is also actuarial evidence that most life insurance money was paid to beneficiaries of homeopathic patients because these people lived longer.[78]
>
> Reprinted with permission of Dana Ullman, from **Discovering Homeopathy**, published by North Atlantic Books, Berkeley CA. 1991, pg. 43.

Using homeopathic remedies raises the overall level of health because it enables a person to establish an immune response which will prevent disease. The Polio vaccine is an example of homeopathic medicine. It uses a small amount of a known toxin, namely the killed virus, in order to elicit an immune response which makes a person forever immune to the polio virus.

Unlike homeopathy, vaccines contain other harmful ingredients so we recommend avoiding them.

---

[77]   New England Medical Gazette, 1866, pg. 69.

[78]   Transactions of The American Institute of Homeopathy, 1892, pg. 83.

The history of homeopathy begins with the discoveries of its founder, Samuel Hahnemann (1755-1843), a German Physician. Hahnemann first coined the word *homeopathy (homoios* in Greek means "similar," *pathos* means "suffering")* to refer to the pharmacological principle, the law of similars, that is its basis. Actually the law of similars was previously described by Hippocrates and Paracelsus and was utilized by many cultures, including the Mayans, Chinese, Greeks, Native American Indians and Asian Indians,[79] but it was Hahnemann who codified the law into a systematic medical science.

Reprinted with permission of Dana Ullman, from **Discovering Homeopathy**, published by North Atlantic Books, Berkeley CA. 1991, pg. 33.

At a health conference in 1976 Jonas Salk noted that there are basically two ways to heal sick people. First, one can try to control the individual symptoms that the sick person is experiencing; and second, one can try to stimulate the person's own immune and defense systems to enable the body to heal itself. Whereas conventional medicine's allegiance is to the first approach, homeopathy and a wide variety of natural healing systems attempt the latter.

Reprinted with permission of Dana Ullman, from **Discovering Homeopathy**, published by North Atlantic Books, Berkeley CA. 1991, pg. 122.

---

[79]   Sir James George Frazer, **The Golden Bough** (New York: Macmillan, 1992) pgs. 12-42

"A little known fact of history is that homeopathic medicine developed its popularity in both the United States and Europe because of its successes in treating epidemics that raged in the 19th century. In 1849 the homeopaths of Cincinnati claimed that in over a thousand cases of cholera only 3 percent of the patients died."

Reprinted with permission of Dana Ullman, from **Discovering Homeopathy**, published by North Atlantic Books, Berkeley CA. 1991, pg. 126

"Homeopathy offers a different philosophy since its medicines are not simply intended to be antibacterial or antiviral but to stimulate the person's overall resistance to infection. Homeopathic remedies strengthen the organism so that it is more capable of defending itself, and do so without producing the side effects commonly experienced with antibiotics. Such treatment provides a more ecological approach to curing infectious disease, since it aids the body's natural homeostasis without suppressing the organism's inherent self-protective response."

Reprinted with permission of Dana Ullman, from **Discovering Homeopathy**, published by North Atlantic Books, Berkeley CA. 1991, pg. xxix.

Darwin noted that the body automatically raised its temperature when it became infected with germs or viruses in order to kill the invaders. When you have a fever it stimulates macrophages (the body's killer cells that destroy toxins) to rush to the infected area and destroy germs and bacteria. The heat from the fever literally fries the bacteria and harmful microbes.

Darwin felt that this process should not be disturbed since it is a form of natural healing that the body has evolved. Likewise, vomiting and diarrhea are symptoms that confirm that the body is indeed ridding itself of toxins.

Working as an acupressure practitioner I very often notice that on the outside of the skin on top of a knot or tumor there are usually one or more pus-filled pimples. This is an indication that the body is trying to discharge toxins through the skin. I tell my patients to sleep with a cotton ball soaked in 3 percent hydrogen peroxide over it, which will suck the toxins out in many cases.

In many cases, when we interfere with natural body processes like aspirin for fever and pink medicine for diarrhea, we interfere with the body's self-healing mechanisms. Yet there are many things that we can do to help them along.

Taking homeopathic medicines is one of them. Instead of aspirin for headache, take *Aconite, Nux Vomica, Arnica or Belladonna. For diarrhea try* Arsenicum, Cuprum Arsenicosum or *Aconite.*

Homeopathic practice is based on the belief that a microdose of a toxic substance can cure an ailment with similar symptoms to that produced by a large toxic dose of that substance. This means that a homeopath will give you a small dose of some substance (usually a root, mineral or an herb, but not always, but always something natural) that would in large doses cause your ailment.

The small dose evokes the healing response in the body. The microdoses have a bioelectronic charge that acts upon the bioenergetic processes of the body.

No one knows how these therapies work, only that they do. Homeopathy has withstood the test of time. There is no effective treatment in conventional medicine for viruses, but there are homeopathic remedies that work on viruses. After being sickly almost all my life, I am a witness that the therapies actually do work!

After spending 1,000 dollars to treat a bladder infection using conventional (allopathic) doctors, and still with the infection, and another condition created by the antibiotics, on the advice of a friend, I found a quick cure for four dollars and fifty cents at my local homeopathic pharmacy.

Within three days, the burning and pressure were gone. I was sold, and everyone I refer to homeopathic treatment gets great benefit from it, grows to love it and stays with it. If you try homeopathy, so will you! Imagine what you can save in medical costs.

One of the beauties of homeopathic treatment is that it is ancient, natural and inexpensive (usually, a cure can be had for 4 dollars and fifty cents, whereas, if you went to a conventional medical doctor, you might put out 300 dollars for lab tests plus 60-150 dollars for the doctor's fee). You can read a simple book on homeopathy and treat yourself and your family safely.

Take homeopathic medicines for one week at a time unless under the direction of a homeopathic physician.

"Homeopaths conceptualize a "life-force" or "vital force," which they describe as the inherent, underlying, interconnective, self-healing process of the organism. This bioenergetic force is similar to what the Chinese call "chi," the Japanese call "ki,", yogis call "prana," Russian scientists call "bioplasm" and Star Wars characters call "The Force." Homeopaths theorize that this bioenergetic process is sensitive to the submolecular homeopathic medicines. The resonance of the microdose is thought to affect the resonance of the person's life-force."

Reprinted with permission of Dana Ullman, from **Discovering Homeopathy**, published by North Atlantic Books, Berkeley CA. 1991, pg. 15.

"New laboratory research has also showed the beneficial effects of homeopathic medicines on the immune function. The **European Journal of Pharmacology** for instance, published research which showed that a commonly used homeopathic medicine, *Silica*, had dramatic effects on stimulating macrophages. Macrophages, a type of white blood cell that devours dead cells, are an important part of the body's defenses. *Silica* 10c was found to stimulate macrophage activity by as much as 67.5 percent.

New research published in the **International Journal of Immunotherapy** has shown that microdoses used in homeopathy corrected immunological disorders in New Zealand mice. These same researchers also found that microdoses of interferon had immunomodulatory effects on New Zealand mice."

Reprinted with permission of Dana Ullman, from **Discovering Homeopathy**, published by North Atlantic Books, Berkeley CA. 1991, pg. 228.

"Another study published in a respected pharmacology journal showed that *Silica 6c and Silica* 10c had statistically significant effects on stimulating macrophages in mice. (Macrophages are essential parts of the immune system and help destroy foreign particles, bacteria, and other cells.) This evidence showing that homeopathic medicines can be used to stimulate immune responses is of particular importance. A study showing the antiviral activity of homeopathic medicines may have special importance today because of the sudden global increase in serious viral infections. An experiment on chicken embryos showed that eight out of ten homeopathic medicines tested inhibited viruses between 50 and 100 percent."

Reprinted with permission of Dana Ullman, from **Discovering Homeopathy**, published by North Atlantic Books, Berkeley CA. 1991. pg. 64.

"In another article published in *Thorax* the case of a 59-year old man was described. This patient had a type of lung cancer in which the average length of survival if left untreated is six to 17 weeks from the time of diagnosis. However, as the result of homeopathic treatment and the use of the herb mistletoe (Iscador), this patient lived five years seven months after diagnosis."

Reprinted with permission of Dana Ullman, from **Discovering Homeopathy**, published by North Atlantic Books, Berkeley CA. 1991 pg. xviii.

"Homeopaths conceptualize a "life-force" or "vital force," which they describe as the inherent, underlying, interconnective, self-healing process of the organism. This bioenergetic force is similar to what the Chinese call "chi," the Japanese call "ki," yogis call "prana," Russian scientists call "bioplasm" and Star Wars characters call "The Force." Homeopaths theorize that this bioenergetic process is sensitive to the submolecular homeopathic medicines. The resonance of the microdose is thought to affect the resonance of the person's life-force."

Reprinted with permission of Dana Ullman, from **Discovering Homeopathy**, published by North Atlantic Books, Berkeley CA. 1991, pg. 15.

"New laboratory research has also showed the beneficial effects of homeopathic medicines on the immune function. The **European Journal of Pharmacology** for instance, published research which showed that a commonly used homeopathic medicine, *Silica*, had dramatic effects on stimulating macrophages. Macrophages, a type of white blood cell that devours dead cells, are an important part of the body's defenses. *Silica* 10c was found to stimulate macrophage activity by as much as 67.5 percent.

New research published in the **International Journal of Immunotherapy** has shown that microdoses used in homeopathy corrected immunological disorders in New Zealand mice. These same researchers also found that microdoses of interferon had immunomodulatory effects on New Zealand mice."

Reprinted with permission of Dana Ullman, from **Discovering Homeopathy**, published by North Atlantic Books, Berkeley CA. 1991, pg. 228.

"A double-blind experiment was performed on 61 people with varicose veins. Conducted in Germany, this study used a combination of eight homeopathic medicines; *Meliotus* (sweet clover) 1x, *Aesculus* (horse chestnut) 1x, *Carduus marianus* (St. Mary's thistle) 1x, *Arnica* tincture (mountain daisy), *Lycopodium* (club moss) 4x, *Lachesis* (venom of the bushmaster) 4x, and Rutin 1x. The subjects of the experiment were given three doses daily for 24 days. This study measured various objective and subjective symptoms of the patients. The results showed an astounding difference between those patients given the homeopathic medicines and those given the placebo. Those given the homeopathic medicines improved by 44 percent, while those given the placebo deteriorated 18 percent."

Reprinted with permission of Dana Ullman, from **Discovering Homeopathy**, published by North Atlantic Books, Berkeley CA. 1991. pg. xvii.

The beauty of homeopathy is that it provides remedies for both physical as well as emotional problems. Homeopaths believe that any illness is a symptom that there is some imbalance in mind, body or spirit of the organism. Some of the medicines that help emotional problems are: *Chamomile* for irritability, or stomachache following emotional upset; *Ignatia* for grief or helping get over a lost love. *Aconite* is for anxiety and illnesses caused by fright.

If you hold a grudge against someone, your anger can do you in. Hostility makes your brain make the harmful hormones cortisol and epinepherine. Since we were intended to be benevolent, and, when you think about it, it makes life so much easier, you might as well give in and go with the flow and let the good vibes happen. If they don't happen naturally, a little effort from you will make them happen. All you have to do is change your internal conversation with yourself.

How do you do that? You take charge of your brain and steer it in the direction you want it in, instead of allowing it go off on tangents. Instead of backstabbing a co-worker or family member, and adding to the chaos and confusion, why not do what you can to create peace and harmony? Don't go with the normal flow of things the way you have always done in the past.

Do things a little differently, and your life will change dramatically! Try talking problems out with the person you differ with instead of standing back and holding a grudge and taking your anger out on them in little subtle ways. Do you really want to be the kind of person that participates in such petty behavior?

Try compromising. Don't leave hard feelings to fester. The effect really does trickle down, and everyone around the hostility will be affected. Walk a mile in the person's shoes. Homeopathic medicines work for emotional upsets and, unlike the many other drugs on the market, they contain no alcohol, and are never toxic.

These medicines have proved themselves through the test of time. They reestablish health. Food allergies are reduced if not eliminated since homeopathic medicines re-establish the immune system. Please follow the guidelines below when taking homeopathic medicines:

- *Diagnosis should be based on symptoms*
- *Always start with low dosages*
- *Take medicines three times a day, one hour before, or two hours after meals.*
- *Do not drink with medicines*
- *Take for one week at a time, unless recommended by a doctor*

Einstein said that we exist in a minimum of four dimensions, three of them being space and one of them being time. He believed that what happened in our past affected us greatly. He said there is no past and future, only now, and that the present encompassed all time.

Homeopaths have come to realize that when an event shocks the vital force, our chi, then it can disturb the harmonious flow of the organism. This disturbance can lead to disease.

One of the more stressful environments in life that many people grit their teeth and bear is the workplace. Here there are found innumerable aggravating scenarios. Notice when your relationship with someone else does not work it is usually when you can not get them to do, be or act as you want them to, and vice versa.

Notice this: when you feel disgusted with someone, look deep inside yourself and you will see that you are disgusted with them because you hate that same disgusting quality about yourself.

We also usually accuse people of being like we are. How often I have heard someone say, "She's spoiled," or "He's selfish," and I thought with wonder, that's precisely true and stands out about him or her. Next time you find yourself complaining about someone, look deep and you will see that the very trait that you are complaining about is one of your own that you don't like.

If we just sit back and experience people as they are, and enjoy them, and not try to make them into our recipe of how a person is supposed to be, then life could be really cool. But no one can do that. We all expect people to conform to our role-model and live up to our ideals.

And when they don't, that's when the problems begin. Actually, when you think about it realistically, it makes no sense. How can anyone possibly know how we are expecting them to act or be? This is one of the great conundrums in human relationships.

One of the things that helped me decide I did not want to work in an office setting was working in them for twenty years. Some of my worst intolerances were for gossip and the petty innuendoes and crude insensitivities, like gum popping, power struggles, sucking up and the grungies that some people keep going.

I understood more why Europeans think we Americans are crude and crass when I went there. They never chew gum. They mostly don't dress casually. They are almost always on their best behavior. No wonder we look primitive and disgusting to some of them.

What happens in the office is that various conflicts grow out of proportion and are tossed about or left hanging, both deadly ways to deal with conflict. I concluded that people in offices, being sealed off like that from nature in an unnatural environment- -lost the ability to prioritize. Help them? Forget it, for they all know all the answers, same as I did.

An example of the insanity: they had good jobs, did not have to work themselves to death, were well paid, fat and downright lazy, and most of the time all they did was complain or throw sick jokes at each other, when they could have been having fun.

And every time I tried to tell them that they had a choice, that they really had it all if only they could see it, that they could diminish the negative and enhance the positive, they said, "Miss positive, you try to find positive in everything, even disaster." I said, "I do because there is something positive in disaster and its the wisdom you learn."

But having been an unwilling participant in many toxic workplace incidents, I want to point out that these caustic incidents can build up and grow like cancers. *Yes, they can even shock the vital force if they are not resolved.* They can affect one's health greatly.

I have known numerous women who came down with a severe headache every Sunday night. Each time I had to point out that the prospect of returning to work was causing it, and each time, they reluctantly admitted, that yes, the job stress was terrible. They had not associated the two.

The important point being made here is that not just bacteria and viruses cause disease. Stress and stressful situations day in and day out cause it also. When we are under stress or feeling angry our brain makes toxic hormones .

One of the great injustices and in my opinion, crimes that our society commits to young children is: make young children in school sit on the ground and on the floor. On the ground, even on the grass, there are millions of microorganisms waiting for a warm body to live in. The worms, cysts, parasites are there waiting and as soon as the child sits on the ground/floor, they activate, bore through the skin, travel through the bloodstream and start killing the child. IT takes some time for this, because the microbes are very small. Check the Center For Disease Control website. Look up Hookworms, or Ascaris, although there are many others. See the book by Roger Knudson called *FEARSOME FAUNA*, A Field Guide To the Creatures That Live In You. The front cover of the August 2000 Discover Magazine shouts DO PARASITES RULE THE WORLD? Here are some web addresses that will confirm what I am saying: http://www.cdc.gov/ncidod/dpd/parasites/hookworm/factsht hookworm.htm and http://www.cdc.gov/ncidod/diseases/roundwrm/roundwrm. htm. One of the more deadly parasites the children will get will be hookworms. They and many of the other parasites in the soil cause death. These children, by the time they are twenty to thirty years old will be chubby, even obese, and it is from the parasites growing in them. I would like parents to get together and stand up for their children: insist that the school does no make your child sit on the ground or floor. This silent killer of children causes me much grief.

HOW EXCESSIVE STRESS KILLS
YOU SLOWLY

Hans Selye discovered the stress response more than thirty years ago. Since then, researchers have tested and discovered much more about the hazards of stress. The way it works is that when a stressful event begins, it registers on the central nervous system and on a person's physical, emotional and spiritual psyche. This state of alarm is called "fight-or-flight" because it also allows a massive amount of energy to stand by for action. It almost seems as if nature designed this first stage of stress to deal with day-to-day petty annoyances.

For the duration of the stressful situation, our bodies go into a type of code red and our stress mechanisms are turned on. When the event is over, this all gets turned off again. But suppose the stressful episode lasts a month, or three years? If the stress continues, the body goes into the next stage, the stage of resistance. This is when some people turn to relaxants, extra-marital affairs, drugs and alcohol. Some simply bear it out. This second stage can become chronic if it can't be turned of. The biological effects of it can destroy a person.

The effects are:
1. Elevation of blood pressure that could become chronic. High blood pressure causes slow, steady damage to the heart, kidneys and cardiovascular system.
2. Arterial walls tear and clotting elements in the blood increase, causing clogging of the arteries.
3. Blood sugar levels increase, which in turn raise cholesterol.
4. Resistance to disease is lowered because critical white blood cell levels decrease.
5. Stomach acids increase and change the lining of the stomach, which can lead to ulcers and gastrointestinal distress.
6. Joints become inflamed due to stuck fluids because anxiety interferes with the smooth flow of lymph fluids. Neck and shoulders become stiff and achy.
7. The entire body becomes hyperactive, which results in mental and physical exhaustion, insomnia.
8. When adrenalin levels are high for prolonged periods of time, vasopressin raises blood pressure by narrowing arteries.
9. Metabolism is accelerated because a thyrotrophic hormone (TTH) stimulates the thyroid to increase its production. Cortisol, which raises blood sugar, and alters the immune system, is produced.

We were taught at an early age that all our cuts and abrasions must be treated with mercurochrome, hydrogen peroxide, betadine or provodine iodine and then covered to keep dirt and infection out until the skin closed up, and it turns out that treatment is just as important today as it was then.

Have you ever noticed the bacteria that grows in your toilet before you wash them away? One of the things that harms women that they never dream of is this filthy water from the toilet splashing up and getting on or in their genitals. A drop of this filthy water has enough bacteria in it to cause a serious vaginal infection.

To protect yourself lay a couple of squares of toilet paper on top of the water in the toilet and urinate on it. It will keep the water from popping back up on you and causing infections.

After eating, rinse your mouth to remove food particles that are rich sources for bacteria to grow in and cause tooth decay. Rinsing with hydrogen peroxide is even more effective for preventing cavities, especially when you can't brush. Swish it between your teeth. Before bed rinse with baking soda and water.

Never give a child a toothpick. Do not swallow small pieces of toothpicks as they can lodge in the intestines and cause boils, abscesses and much pain and agony.

When gardening, do not put your bare hands in the dirt as parasites can bore through your skin and make residence in your body, robbing you of important nutritional reserves and health.

I heard a news report which stated that the body fluids of a person with AIDS have recently been reclassified by The Center For Disease Control as one of the most toxic substances on earth, particularly if you contaminate a cut or abrasion on the skin with them.

Chapter 19

ABOUT OXYGEN, THE
MOST HEALING
SUBSTANCE ON EARTH

I would not be here writing this book and sharing this information with you if my ex-husband had not recommended I start taking oxygen internally for my illness. I would be dead. I successfully cured myself of some chronic diseases after taking ten drops of 3 percent food grade hydrogen peroxide in a 10-12 ounce glass of juice three times a day. I now simply swish either the 3 percent food grade or the regular 3 percent around in my mouth, allow it to foam and spit it out or squirt one squirt into a glass of juice. This oxygenates my entire body and has kept me well since I started taking it.

I had Systemic Chronic Candidiasis, which caused me to be weak, dizzy, achy, irrational, anxious, constipated, bloated, sensitive to odors, especially molds and perfumes, suffering with migraines and food addictions, unbearable back pain, chronic yeast infections, depression, irrational irritability, acne, migraine, and I caught everything that came along. I thought I was losing my mind and dying at the same time.

I was terrified at the thought of drinking small amounts of food grade hydrogen peroxide, but I felt I was dying and did not have much to lose. My ex-husband, a scientist whom I have a lot of respect for, assured me that as soon as the hydrogen peroxide went into my body the atoms of hydrogen dropped off and what remained was pure oxygen which would bind to harmful substances and destroy them.

He said the oxygen then went to work like a SWAT team after a group of terrorists to annihilate foreign matter, free radicals,[80] toxins, parasites and especially yeast, bacteria, viruses, and oxygenated the blood, thus, nourishing it,

---

[80]   Free radicals do their damage by destroying tissue when they steal electrons from proteins, nucleic acids and fats. Their damage is one of the leading causes of aging and disease. They are found abundantly in stale oils. Taking oxygen as described in this book destroys them.

and the body all at the same time. He said none of the body's good bacteria would be destroyed, only the bad, and he guaranteed me that it would not harm me. He knew I had been taking nystatin for five years for candida and it had only helped marginally, but wasn't really getting rid of the organisms. He said taking oxygen would get rid of them once and for all. But I felt something else was wrong with me, that I could not be feeling so weak and sick unless I was dying.

Then one week after I started on the oxygen, my new doctor confirmed that the back pain was from lung cancer. During those days, I must have gone to twenty or thirty doctors trying to find out what was wrong with me. As he went over the course of therapy for my kind of cancer: surgical removal of the primary infected area with radiation therapy afterwards to make sure the cancer was all gone and, possibly, chemotherapy, I stopped listening, for I knew I was not strong enough to go through with any of those procedures. Also, I had seen some of my friends and family go though this torturous course of therapy and die, usually shortly after the surgery.

I thought, I'm going to find another way to cure myself. I thought about my divorce the year before as the cause for the cancer. I had been unbearably miserable over it. I remembered Freud had said long ago that the mind causes illness and can cure it. I knew I had to cure myself because I had too much to live for. My determination to live is part of why I survived.

I noticed two weeks after I started taking the oxygen though, that I could concentrate again. I had not realized how much my ability to concentrate had deteriorated. Then, a miracle happened two weeks after that, I started gaining my strength back! You never really know how sick you are until you start getting better.

Sickness is something you sort of sink into like quicksand. I was ill to the point that I worked; I went to work everyday, felt miserable all day but propped myself up for work. Then every evening when I came home, I crashed. I was often too exhausted to even eat. And the exhaustion was getting worse.

I never went back to the doctor who diagnosed my cancer. I discovered a homeopathic medicine for lung cancer, *Viscum Album* 10c. I took it faithfully with oxygen, used Herbal Lotion on the cancer and it went away completely.

There is nothing on earth more exhilarating than finding out you're going to live after you thought you were dying for sure. Even now, I appreciate every minute. I appreciate being on earth. I appreciate the power of my mind and its healing abilities most profoundly. Suppose I'd had this conversation with myself: I've got cancer and I'm going to die. Had I not fought, I'm convinced I would not be here now.

Our conversations with ourselves are very important. Three of the most important reasons I had that conversation with myself that saved my life are my mother, Freud and the Lifespring Basic Awareness Training. All coached me on attaining the impossible. And I have learned that nothing is impossible.

Coming so close to being a corpse or a bed or ashes has greatly intensified my appreciation for life. Once you think about what is at the end for all of us, you can go and enjoy life fully and with abandon, knowing that every breath could have been missed. Knowing that one day you will be a corpse or a pile of ashes can make now a wonderful experience. Because life is precious. Think of the conflicts as a chance for growth.

As I learned while studying Hinduism, everything happens for a reason. If I had not had all that illness, I never would have started taking oxygen, and thus, experience the level of health that I experience today. Let me tell you that when you are sick, your mind does not really function normally. Nothing is really comforting except getting rid of he pain and sickness.

As my health improved I read all I could find about oxygen therapy and homeopathy. I found some interesting studies claiming that both cured people of AIDS, cancer, MS, Candidiasis, arthritis and many other conditions. Funny but had I not gotten the disease, I would not have discovered the cure, which I have shared with hundreds since and everyone survived.

People with AIDS, cancer, arthritis, candida, or any kind of weakness or debility, anyone who has gone barefoot or slept with pets, or suspected of having parasitic infection or weak immune system have benefitted from taking *Silica* 10c, *Carbo vegetabilis*, Black Walnut and oxygen as described here. I get reports of amazing, effective results from those who read **Oxygen Therapies** and use oxygen to treat their illness. Oxygen has not only been discovered to destroy toxins, diseases, viruses and foreign matter in the blood, it also nourishes and sustains the cells. Oxygen is the greatest thing! It saved my life. It can save yours too.

Following is one of the first things I read before starting to take oxygen, then, an updated version. **Hydrogen Peroxide Facts** by Kurt W. Donsbach, D.C. Ph.D. © by Dr. Donsbach. Reprinted with permission.

Hydrogen Peroxide Facts

Kurt W. Donsbach, D.C., N.D., Ph.D.

There have been many incorrect statements regarding the ingestion of hydrogen peroxide and now, magnesium peroxide. I would like to address these so that you as a patient will not be misled and stop using a potentially beneficial product.

Myth #1: Any of the peroxides destroy friendly bacteria in the gut and require that you reintroduce fresh bacteria constantly if you are using the peroxide on a regular basis. The proof offered was that when you put hydrogen peroxide into a yogurt culture, the resultant yogurt was weak and watery.

FACTS: THE FRIENDLY BACTERIA IN THE GUT ARE AEROBIC, MEANING THEY LIVE AS AN OXYGEN-USING ORGANISM. If you want the opinion of the bible of bacteriology, check this out in *Bergey's Manual of Systematic Bacteriology* or *Clinical Diagnosis by Laboratory Methods* by Todd & Sanford. The addition of extra oxygen to the yogurt culture could have altered other factors in the milk used in the culture, rather than destroying the lactobacillus. The reference used by the writer was conspiciously lacking bacteria counts before and after the addition of the hydrogen peroxide! The truth is you help, not hinder, lactobacillus with H_2O_2.

Myth #2: Oral ingestion of hydrogen peroxide promotes the growth of various viruses, including what has been called the EBV virus, the HIV virus and others.

FACTS: HYDROGEN PEROXIDE IS CAPABLE OF DESTROYING EACH AND EVERY ONE OF THESE VIRUSES IN LABORATORY TESTS. This does not necessarily mean that the same action occurs in the body, but it is a pretty good indicator. THE MOST IMPORTANT FACT REGARDING THIS ALLEGATION IS NOT WHETHER OR NOT HYDROGEN PEROXIDE KILLS OR STIMULATES A VIRUS, BUT HOW HYDROGEN PEROXIDE IS HANDLED BY THE BODY WHEN IT IS ABSORBED FROM THE GUT. What actually occurs is that the instant hydrogen peroxide crosses the intestinal barrier and enters the blood stream, the enzyme catalase splits the compound into water and free radical oxygen. This takes one molecule of catalase for every 10,000 molecules of hydrogen peroxide and uses up about 1/10,000 of a second. In approximately another 1/10,000 of a second you will see one free radical oxygen (O_1) join another free radical oxygen to form stable oxygen (O_2). Since this all takes approximately 1/5,000 of a second, when does the hydrogen peroxide have time to enter the circulatory channels and end up in the T cells where the HIV virus proliferates? Obviously it doesn't. THIS IS ALSO THE ANSWER TO THE CLAIM THAT FREE RADICAL OXYGEN WILL CAUSE CELLULAR DAMAGE. THE FREE RADICAL OXYGEN HAS AN EXTREMELY SHORT LIFE IN THE BLOOD STREAM ONLY AND NEVER GETS CLOSE TO CELLS!

The following excerpt from A Progress Report, Oxygen Therapy by Walter Grotz is reprinted with permission of Mr. Grotz, formerly of ECHO of Delano, MN.

The information contained in this booklet is for educational purposes only. It is not to be considered medical advice, diagnostic or prescriptive. See your doctor for qualified health care.

41 million Americans have serious arthritis, 20 million have herpes, 13 million have serious diabetes. This is 74 million or over one third of our population and we have only covered three diseases. At the beginning of this century we were one of the healthiest nations on this earth. We are the wealthiest, but far from being the healthiest.

Some of the reasons for this are that our air, water and food are not what they were 75 to 100 years ago. We have polluted the air, we need additives for our water to make it safe to drink, and our food has lost its trace elements, long leached from our soils. We now must use supplements to help supply what has been lost. One of these supplements is oxygen.

Oxygen is the most abundant element on earth. It comprises 45.6% of the earth's crust and 20.95% of dry air. It is one of the most vital and necessary elements to support life. Oxygen is so vital to good health that hospitals have it installed in patient's rooms. All rescue units, ambulances and life support systems are equipped with it. Without oxygen you can live only a few minutes.

Through his research efforts, Dr. Edward Carl Rosenow (1875 - 1966) worked out the causes of some 35 diseases and was the author of 450 medical papers. Dr. Rosenow developed a technique by which microorganisms in the body could possibly be eliminated or controlled. The hydrogen peroxide program is a method of taking oxygen into the body to possibly eliminate or control these mircroorganisms.

His basic tenet was that we live in an ocean of microorganisms. The body is like a world. In the world of the body are millions of microorganisms — little creatures each seeking their own habitat, food and environment. Just as animals in our world live in different climates, eat different foods, multiply, prey upon others, infect, go through metamorphosis, pollute streams, so these little microorganisms invade our bodies and seek out their proper habitats. These microorganisms do the following:

— gnaw away at the joints (inflammatory arthritis)
— Give off calcium waste matter that cements bones together
— lodge in liver and kidneys, and with their bite form stones
— live in the very lining of the arteries and leave their hard deposit on the walls of the arteries
— cling to the lining in the nervous system and short-circuit some of the electronics in the central computer of the brain
— attack cells and enter them, building cocoons around the stricken cell; thus cutting off the blood supply and causing the cell to lose its specific function, so that it can only live and multiply into cancerous tumors.

One of the simplest sources of this healing oxygen is in hydrogen peroxide. Hydrogen peroxide traces back through to the origin of time. It was first reported by the French chemist Louis-Jacques Thenard in 1818, who named it eau oxygenee. It is very natural; it is found in traces as rain and snow (McGraw-Hill Encyclopedia of Science & Technology 5th Edition, p. 747). In 1863 Meissner proved its presence in the rainwater collected during thunder storms and this has been corroborated by others (Journal of the American Medical Association, Vol. X, No. 9, March 3, 1888) It gets into our rain and snow from the ozone layer high in the earth's atmosphere. It can also be created in the atmosphere when ultraviolet light strikes oxygen in the presence of moisture. Ozone (O_3) is free oxygen (O_2) plus an extra atom of oxygen. This extra atom of oxygen splits off very easily, and does so when it comes in contact with water. Water (H_2O) now becomes hydrogen peroxide (H_2O_2).

Compared to chlorine, bacterial and viral disinfection with ozone is up to 5000 times more rapid. (McGraw-Hill Encyclopedia of Science & Technology 5th Edition, P. 728) This is why many cities in Europe use ozone and hydrogen peroxide in their drinking waters. Many brands of bottled water that you buy in this country have been ozonated for your protection.

Hydrogen peroxide is found in fresh fruits and vegetables; some of it comes from rain and some of it is manufactured in the photosynthesis process. (Gen. Biochemistry Furton & Sommonds, p. 338) If we were to eat fresh fruits and vegetables in their raw state, we would get this healing oxygen into our bodies.

We tested human mother's milk and found it contains a good amount of natural hydrogen peroxide. Colostrum milk (first milk secreted after birth) has an even stronger hydrogen peroxide content. In testing natural spring waters, we found the spring water at Lourdes, France contained the strongest amount of hydrogen peroxide in its natural form.

Since 1966 there have been over 6000 medical articles published about hydrogen peroxide. They do not all concern human beings and they are not all positive. An article on the internal injection of hydrogen peroxide appeared in The Lancet Feb. 21, 1920 (Influenzal Pneumonia: The Intravenous Injection of Hydrogen Peroxide pp. 432-433) An article on external use appeared in Hautarzt 12:425 Sept. 1961 Germany (On a Simple and Painless Treatment of Warts). In 1983 there were over 100 articles published on the subject of hydrogen peroxide. From 1880 to 1904 Charles Marchand published eighteen books on the subject of hydrogen peroxide and ozone. A listing of some of these articles appears later in this booklet. The complete articles can be found in medical libraries.

The Food & Drug Administration (FDA) in Federal Regulation Vol. 46 Number 6 Jan. 9, 1981, in effect gave the food industry a green light to use hydrogen peroxide in the "Aseptic" packaging process. The FDA has further ruled that hydrogen peroxide can be used in the processing of cheese and related cheese products (part 133), eggs and egg products (part 160), and as an antimicrobial agent in whey processing. They have also ruled it to be used in cleaning and healing mouth injuries. It is used in milk in 45 countries around the world. A good article on the "Aseptic" process for milk can be found in Trailer Life Nov. 1981 pp. 51-52.

NOTE: THE FDA HAS NOT APPROVED OF THE USE OF THE PURGING SCHEDULES OR OF THE DRINKING OF HYDROGEN PEROXIDE INTERNALLY. THOSE WHO CHOOSE TO DO SO, DO IT OF THEIR OWN VOLITION. THE INFORMATION IS PASSED ALONG FOR RESEARCH AND EDUCATIONAL PURPOSES ONLY AND THOSE WHO CHOOSE TO USE IT ASSUME ALL RESPONSIBILITY PERSONALLY.

Two purging schedules follow for the experimental oral hydrogen peroxide program. The first one uses 6% food grade hydrogen peroxide and the second one uses 3%. With either program, A .5% SOLUTION SHOULD NOT BE EXCEEDED. STRONG SOLUTIONS OF HYDROGEN PEROXDE MAY CAUSE INJURY, ILLNESS OR MAY EVEN BE FATAL.

DO NOT USE THE HYDROGEN PEROXIDE PROGRAM IF YOU HAVE AN ORGAN TRANSPLANT AS IT MAY POSSIBLY CAUSE REJECTION.

PURGING SCHEDULE FOR 6% FOOD GRADE H_2O_2

Tolerance levels seem to vary for persons using hydrogen peroxide, but these guidelines seem generally satisfactory. The 6% food grade hydrogen peroxide concentrate MUST BE DILUTED in water or other liquid before using. It is preferable to use distilled water for this dilution.

Drink this mixture on an empty stomach. It is usually taken ONE HOUR BEFORE OR THREE HOURS AFTER A MEAL. Some prefer to take the solution just before going to bed, but you can work out your own system.

ADD QUANTITIES SHOWN TO 5 - 8 OUNCES DISTILLED OR SPRING WATER, MILK, VEGETABLE OR FRUIT JUICES; no sugar, alcoholic or carbonated-type beverages are to be used, nor fresh pressed carrot juice or bananas that have been blended. There is an enzyme in fresh pressed carrot juice and/or bananas that breaks down H_2O_2 into water and oxygen. (You may have bananas or fresh pressed carrot juice at other times of the day.) When reaching higher levels of hydrogen peroxide, more water or juice may be taken as needed. DO NOT INGEST THE PURE 6% FOOD GRADE HYDROGEN PEROXIDE.

1st day	½ teaspoon
2nd day	1 teaspoon
3rd day	1½ teaspoons
4th day	2 teaspoons
5th day	2½ teaspoons
6th through 12th day	2 teaspoons (3 times daily)
13th through 19th day	2 teaspoons (twice daily)
20th through 27th day	2 teaspoon per day

Then, two teaspoons every other day for a week.

Then cut back to 1 teaspoon every other day; or else take about ½ teaspoon daily as may be necessary. ALWAYS judge your own particular requirements.

CAUTION: If any strong solution of hydrogen peroxide concentrate is spilled on the skin, flush the skin immediately with water. Fingertips may whiten temporarily.

KEEP HYDROGEN PEROXIDE CONCENTRATE OUT OF THE REACH OF CHILDREN AT ALL TIMES. DO NOT TRANSFER HYDROGEN PEROXIDE OF ANY STRENGTH TO AN IMPROPERLY LABELED OR UNLABELED CONTAINER.

Store 6% or 3% food grade hydrogen peroxide in a cool, dry place. Refrigeration is not necessary.

PURGING SCHEDULE FOR 3% FOOD GRADE H_2O_2

The simple schedule for mixing 3% food grade hydrogen peroxide is: one part of 3% solution of hydrogen peroxide with five parts of distilled water, giving you a .5% solution of hydrogen peroxide. Get a gallon of distilled water; take out 20 ounces of water and replace with 20 ounces of 3% food grade hydrogen peroxide and you will have the proper solution.

Drink this mixture on an empty stomach. It is usually taken one hour before or three hours after a meal. One method of taking this mixture is to do so just before going to bed, but work out your own system.

1 oz. the 1st day	5 ozs. 3 times a day for 7 days.
2 ozs. the 2nd day	5 ozs. 2 times a day for 7 days.
3 ozs. the 3rd day	5 ozs. once a day for 7 days.
4 ozs. the 4th day	5 ozs. once every other day for 7 days.
5 ozs. the 5th day	5 ozs. once every third day for 7 days.
THEN TRY	5 ozs. once every fourth day for 7 days.

If you find that the above amounts are more than you can tolerate, then back off on the amount of intake until you feel you are at a comfortable level. Then stay at that level until you get the results you are looking for. One thing to remember is that persistence pays off.

If your condition is severe, stay on 5 ounces of the .5% solution twice a day as long as you think it is necessary.

If you are on supplements, treat them the same as food, taking hydrogen peroxide one hour before or three hours after food or supplements. If you are on a medication, consult your doctor.

If you have a weak stomach, try 1 oz. of 3% hydrogen peroxide in 5 ozs. of milk, vegetable or fruit juice, non-alcoholic or non-carbonated beverage.

Deep breathing of fresh air, along with exercise, is very important.

Hydrogen peroxide is sold in drug stores and grocery stores as an antiseptic; it has been around for many years. It is called Oxygen Water in many countries around the world. In Spain it is called Agua Oxigenada, in Italy Acqua Ossigenata, in France Eau Oxigenee. In the United States we call it Hydrogen Peroxide (H_2O_2).

Have You And Your Cats Had Your Oxygen Today? by Pat McKay is reprinted by permission. © 1993 by Pat McKay.

Have You And Your Cats Had Your Oxygen Today?

by Pat McKay
Animal Nutritionist

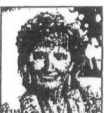

Pat McKay is the author of Reigning Cats And Dogs

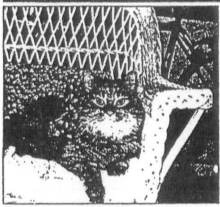

Benefiting fom oxygen: Butterscotch

Oxygen therapy? Who would ever think of it as a healing therapy. We take for granted that we have sufficient oxygen available to us at all times. Oxygen, the colorless, odorless gas that combines with nitrogen and other gases to form our atmosphere, is in trouble. Decades ago the air engulfing our planet was 38 percent oxygen. Now it ranges from as low as 10 percent in many of our cities to 20 percent under the best of country conditions.

In addition to oxygen-deprivation from the environment, our oxygen levels, and our cats', can drop because of injury or disease. Low body temperature can be due to an oxygen-impoverished blood supply. Cancer, AIDS, feline leukemia, arthritis, viruses, harmful bacteria and fungi are anaerobic and thrive in an oxygen-starved system. Antibiotics are detrimental because they destroy the friendly bacteria which produce hydrogen peroxide. It is easy to see why any condition or ailment can be aided and/or prevented by taking O_2.

Extra oxygen can be obtained from fresh, raw fruits and vegetables because they contain hydrogen peroxide that the body converts to stabilized oxygen. Oxygen can also be taken just like vitamins.

Homozon, the brand that I prefer, is a magnesium-based product in powdered form that provides stabilized oxygen which speeds digestion, facilitates removal of diseased and dying cells and cleanses the system by oxidizing old fecal matter without harming the mucosa or lining of the intestines.

A few months ago a cat named Butterscotch had a serious liver condition, was constipated and had the worst backup of hairballs I had ever encountered. Because this cat's system was in such a weakened condition we had to use something very gentle and be careful not to overburden her liver or kidneys, so I suggested Homozon. After three doses of O_2 this cat was on her way to happy littering. Over a three-month period, Butterscotch eliminated twenty-eight inches of impacted hairballs that had been in her system for months, maybe years.

Overweight cats do well on O_2 because it speeds digestion, helps assimilate nutritents more efficiently, improves elimination and provides more energy, all of which builds muscle instead of fat. Underweight cats gain weight for all the same reasons. Just as constipation or diarrhea is often a symptom of the same problems, so is being underweight or overweight.

People and animals, even if they appear to be healthy, should be taking some form of oxygen on a regular, or at least occasional, basis. A cat should take from 1/16 teaspoon once every few days to 1/2 teaspoon twice a day, depending on the animal's size and degree of health. The powder can be mixed with a little bit of raw meat and given like a trea;. The action of Homozon lasts approximately twenty minutes so be sure it is eaten immediately to get the full benefit of the oxygen. If your cat won't eat a raw meat treat right away, the Homozon can be dissolved in a teaspoon of purified water and given with a syringe or glass dropper.

How much you give and how often you give it is determined by watching the consistency of the stools. When the stools become soft like mashed potatoes, yogurt or pea

You can find this product on ebay search for oxy cleanse

Some Parts of the following Condensed from **selfhacked.com**

https://www.selfhacked.com/blog/hydrogen-water/

The Health Benefits of Hydrogen Water- it is an Antioxidant and Prevents Brain Damage. Molecular hydrogen (H2) can protect cells and tissues from oxidative damage by selectively reducing reactive oxygen species (ROS). Most cost effective way to obtain it is to buy Patrick Flanagan's MegaHydrate online for about $29. Many companies now sell various versions of it for double and more. *To make a super healing drink that cures many illnesses, mix one crystallized oxygen pill without herbs with one Megahydrate by dissolving in a quart of water and drink. This concoction has made miracles happen.* Unlike other antioxidants, H2 has the unique capability of crossing cell membranes and targeting organelles such as the mitochondria and nucleus. Proven to help prevent the development of Parkinson's disease in an experiment on rats, reduced oxidative stress and prevented cognitive impairment associated with dementia and Parkinson's disease .

Prevented both the development and progression of neural degeneration, and also suppressed neuronal loss in another Parkinson's disease mice study. Reduces neurotoxic damage. There were also no adverse effects from hydrogen water at high doses (1000 mL/day) .2) Hydrogen Water May Improve Mood Disorders.

Restored the natural growth of brain cells in mice. Because antidepressants increase adult neurogenesis, hydrogen water may be used for improving depression and some mental disorders. Suppresses Inflammation, relieved early rheumatoid arthritis, achieved remission and 20% of subjects became symptom-free.

Reduces Muscle Fatigue, Motor Deficits, and Muscle Degeneration. Reduced lactic acid build-up during heavy exercise in young adults and decreased muscle fatigue and enhances mitochrondrial function. It improves a wide variety of diseases and it can save your life.

Reprinted with permission from Ed McCabe. Ed is the author of "O₂xygen Therapies". Copyright 1990.

Ozone is not smog — Ozone is good and natural
by Ed McCabe

Ozone is one of the most beneficial substances on this planet, and the BAD science you hear quoted on the news every night is causing you to subconsciously be afraid of nature, and therefore, a part of life itself. They tell you that somehow hydrogen plus nitrogen equals ozone. $H + N = O_3$? Not on this planet it doesn't!

What is ozone? Simply, oxygen. Three atoms of nature's oxygen. It exists in a very active form for about 30 minutes before breaking down into two atoms of regular oxygen - by giving up one atom of singlet oxygen.

Where does ozone come from? Nature. And nature is efficient. The new growth in the forests, the trees, the grass on your front lawn, and the plankton in the ocean are continually creating oxygen. As you read this, this oxygen is rising up into the atmosphere to where the ozone layer is. In the region of the ozone layer, our rising oxygen is bombarded by the sun's photochemical energy in the form of ultraviolet (UV) rays. This UV energy bombardment changes the oxygen from O_2 -two atoms of stable oxygen, into O_3 - three atoms of unstable active oxygen. We call this pure form of oxygen "Ozone." This is all part of the natural process of life on this living biosphere called earth. The chemical formula for this is $3O_2 > UV > 2O_3$.

Being heavier than the oxygen in the atmosphere, this newly created Ozone falls back to earth, eventually giving up one atom of oxygen, changing back to O_2, and is immediately replaced by more rising oxygen which is also soon changed into ozone by the sun. The ozone falls to earth and is all around us purifying our water and air, decomposing bacteria, molds and fungi. It is the fresh smell of laundry dried outdoors in the country. It is the fresh air at a clean seashore, and the sweet smell in the air after a lightning storm. Lightning, also possessing photochemical energy, creates ozone as well. At least this is how our world was operating until man started ruining it.

Ozone has always been with us in nature, and the fact that ozone gives off that single oxygen atom is a significant factor in life, in medicine, and in toxic waste cleanup technology. Thousands of physicians in Europe have been using ozone as a medical treatment for over 50 years, and the use of ozone in medicine is starting to finally catch on here in the U.S.

How is it used in medicine? This O_3 Ozone is not as stable as regular O_2 oxygen because it has that extra atom of O_1 attached to it. Ozone will readily give up this extra atom of O_1 and revert back to stable oxygen again. This giving off of the O_1 is the reason why ozone has been used in medicine. It has been proven extensively that O_1 will kill bacteria, viruses, fungi and molds by attaching to them and oxidizing and eliminating them. Oxidizing means to burn without giving off light or heat. These bacteria, etcetera, are lower life form organisms, and are mostly anaerobic. That means they can't live around activated oxygen. Doctors using the proper concentrations and correct medical protocols have achieved substantial positive clinical results with ozone. Far from being a poison, ozone, when used properly, has been shown repeatedly to kill pathogens - yet not hurt normal cells. This is because disease causing pathogens do not have any strong enzyme coatings to protect them - as do all the higher life forms like us. For example, pure ozone is available to purify all our country's stored blood supplies. There is no reason why people have had to come home from the hospital with AIDS or hepatitis from blood transfusions. European doctors and respected NY University researchers all state that ozone has been used to eliminate AIDS in humans, animals and blood tests. Without any side effect. Why don't we see this on TV? Why isn't it being used?

Breathing ozonated air or drinking ozonated water (at the safe legal concentration that are already laid out by the government) are two ways of getting activated oxygen into your body. Did you ever drink clean water just downstream from a waterfall and feel invigorated? That was because the water had tumbled over the rocks, thinned out, and absorbed oxygen/ozone from the air. Other methods being explored medically in the U.S. are rectal ozone insufflation, ozone autohemotherapy, and intravenous ozone infusions. All these methods require the use of pure medical grade ozone. Being blatantly non toxic, these methods of killing viruses and bacteria in humans have been in use in European medicine for over 50 years.

Crystal Oxygen is reprinted with permission of Boundary Waters, PO Box 26173, Minneapolis, MN 55425

EVERYTHING YOU MAY EVER HAVE WANTED TO KNOW ABOUT

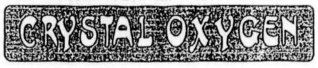

OXYGEN is the primary element in the lives of the entire animal and vegetable kingdoms. Without it, the process of combustion, for example, could not occur. As you know...there is no survival without oxygen!

The air we breathe is a gaseous form of OXYGEN. Besides oxygen, air also supports water vapor and, unfortunately, all forms of pollutants.

Air is not the only source of OXYGEN; fruits, vegetables, and water also take up oxygen. It is available also in BEE PRODUCTS. Oceans have a lot of oxygen...and oxygen is what gives garlic its healthy punch!

But if that wondrous clove of garlic, or any raw food for that matter, is sauteed, cooked, *or processed in any way*...its oxygen is lost.

Joggers and aerobic dancers overcome the lack of OXYGEN in foods by filling their lungs with as much air as possible. Still, in all their ups and downs and running around, their blood oxygen levels may only increase to around 90%...and what about those pollutants the lungs absorb?

There is much to be said about OXYGEN--volumes! There is also a great deal to be said about its taste. Where it is true that HYDROGEN PEROXIDE is an excellent source of OXYGEN, some people, because of its taste, have difficulty taking it in spite of oxygen's benefits. CRYSTAL OXYGEN offers a positive alternative to this dilemma.

That 'taste' has been overcome in some flavored products, but the cost for a month's supply is not a fair trade-off for a pleased palate. CRYSTAL OXYGEN, on the other hand, has overcome both taste and the *trade-offs* of flavored hydrogen peroxide. CRYSTAL OXYGEN is a dry form of HP which is purified through four processes of distillation. It is so pure it becomes CRYSTALLIZED. Although it is packed in capsules with complementary herbs, the BIG PLUS in these capsules is the Oxygen...it raises the BLOOD/OXYGEN level. How much? More than if you were to jog or do aerobic dancing!!

How important is OXYGEN?

Dr. Warburg said it in the early thirties: "...healthy cells thrive on oxygen...or they become cancerous cells from the lack of oxygen..." For this discovery he won the Nobel prize. Oxygen to a healthy cell is like an electrically charged screen door to flies: a virus, like a fly, cannot penetrate these defenses.

The health related properties of oxygen were well known as far back as 1880. A book, *The Therapeutical Applications of Using Hydrazone and Glycozone*, which discusses these properties, was published in 1904 by Dr. Marchand, a chemist. It records the prescribing of oxygen by medical doctors for a variety of diseases. The book is replete with testimonials. Both hydrazone and glycozone consist of superior grades of HYDROGEN PEROXIDE! Grade depends on purity and percent of solution of– OXYGEN.

Doctors, then and now, found that OXYGEN works n three ways: it dissolves excessive deposits of plaque, calculus, and cholesterol in arteries, joints and fine capillaries; it is a selective antibiotic harmful only to health robbing anaerobic bacteria; and it helps maintain a cell's immunity.

Since 1982, hundreds of thousands have re-discovered the properties of OXYGEN in HYDROGEN PEROXIDE, an inexpensive, naturally occurring chemical. Inexpensive, because all it is is WATER and OXYGEN!

---

*Oxygen, A Key
Ingredient For Longevity
and A High Quality Of
Health*

Oxygen is one of the most essential elements for health. It is contained in every cell of our bodies and necessary for every process that occurs in the body. It is so essential that we cannot live more than a few minutes without it. One of the key reasons why exercise is hailed as the fountain of youth is because exercise oxygenates the body. When we sit for hours, out blood congeals. This is dangerous and can lead to strokes and heart attacks. Exercise oxygenates and thins the blood to a safer consistency. One of the reasons why smokers are urged to take vitamin C is because vitamin C oxygenates the cells, and smoking robs the body of oxygen.

Studies have shown that cells deprived of oxygen for short periods of time quickly became malignant. When the cells were again given sustained oxygen, the malignancy was reversed. Since cancer cells cannot live in the presence of large amounts of oxygen, for it is anaerobic (only thrives in an oxygen-free environment) oxygen effectively burns them up. Anyone who knows anything about the body or biology knows the importance of oxygen to the health of cells.

What Dr. Donsbach says proves that the body only benefits from the addition of oxygen, since it plays an important factor in dissolving cancer-causing free radicals. When there is a deficiency of oxygen, malignant cells can start to form, as the following article explains.

Measured Deep Breathing/Meditation has 141 Known Benefits

One of the most important being that it **fills the body with oxygen**. It has been reported that people in India heal themselves of cancer with meditation. Every night I get in bed, say my prayers, then meditate until I fall asleep. Benefits include *slowing aging, mastering stress, great sleep, weight loss, boost serotonin, faster healing, synchronizes the brain*. See all of them here:

https://eocinstitute.org/meditation/141-benefits-of-meditation/?
gclid=EAIaIQobChMIzaHeiqPw2gIV0QOGCh2f-wE4EAAYASAAEgKOo_D_BwE

Oxygen has been taken in various forms to purge, clean out and oxygenate the body. It is also known for destroying germs, viruses, bacteria, foreign matter, and toxins in the body.

Oxygen has never hurt anyone who took it according to the specifications in **Oxygen Therapies** enclosed here. *Oxygen can be harmful if taken in improperly high dosages.*

To learn more about the value of taking oxygen for curing diseases, call or write:

International Bio-Oxidative Medicine Foundation, PO Box 13205, Oklahoma City, OK 73113-1205 phone 405-478-4266 (IBOM)

To order oxygen, contact: Boundary Waters, PO Box 26173, Minneapolis, MN 55426 phone 612-823-9236.

Following is an order form from Boundary Waters for ordering oxygen in the various forms.

PINTS
$6.00 ea.
Case of 12 pints $48.00

QUARTS
$9.00 ea.
Case of 4 quarts $28.00

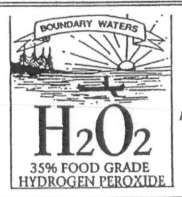
BOUNDARY WATERS
H_2O_2
35% FOOD GRADE
HYDROGEN PEROXIDE

DRUM QUANTITIES AVAILABLE.

PLEASE CALL OR WRITE FOR QUOTE.

NEW!
CRYSTAL OXYGEN
Each cap is equal to 9 to 10 drops of 35% food grade H_2O_2.

180 capsules..........$21
90 capsules..........$11.50

DR. DONSBACH'S SUPEROXY PLUS ALOE VERA
$16.00/Quart

Shipping Included.
Please send check or money order.
Street address needed for U.P.S.

BOUNDARY WATERS H_2O_2
P.O. BOX 26173 • Minneapolis, MN 55426 phone 612-822-5696.

People report that they notice a difference in their energy level after taking oxygen for a few weeks. Little aches and pains melt away. Mine certainly did. I was told to take ten or less drops of 3 percent food grade hydrogen peroxide in a glass of juice three times per day.

That dosage has worked for me and keeps me well to this day. I put the ten drops of 3 percent food grade in fruit juice or a full glass of juice and drink it, or swish it around in my mouth and spit it out.

For crystallized oxygen in pill form I was told to take it one hour before, or two hours after a meal. If you choose not to take food grade hydrogen peroxide, you can often get three 16 ounce bottles of regular 3 percent hydrogen peroxide at the supermarket or drug store for a dollar.

I experimented taking oxygen in this form for one year, although it is not advocated because of the 0.001 percent phosphoric acid used to preserve it. I did not notice any difference. It worked the same with no detectable harmful side effects. I know some people will not go to the trouble to order the food grade.

The important thing is that you try this therapy, for it can add years to anyone's life because it helps increase energy and health. Once you try it, even for a week, you will be hooked, for it will make you feel better than you have felt in a long time. If you elect to take oxygen this way, it has proved to be perfectly safe. Just squirt it in your mouth, allow it to foam for a minute and spit it out.

The oxygen is absorbed through the cells, through the neck and throat and will oxygenate your entire body. Gradually work up to taking it this way two or three times a day.

Cancer cannot grow in the presence of oxygen. This simple fact can save millions of people from cancer if they would just test it. Oxygen effectively burns cancer out. The main cause of cancer and its cure is so simple. Since our earth is so much more polluted now we get 5-20 percent less oxygen from the air then we used to.

Add to that the fact of a sedentary lifestyle of sitting for eight hours at work, and three hours a day watching television. Then there are the seven or eight hours of sleep. That is eighteen hours of inactivity and if there is no exercise day after day, the blood congeals and thickens. Add the factor of a poor diet and you can see how disease begins to develop.

Oxidizers have proved to oxygenate the blood and contribute greatly to health, but especially so for sedentary people. They can dissolve harmful agents and prevent a multitude of diseases in the body. They zap pathogens and foreign matter in the blood. They help stop the body from aging. They oxidize and empower the blood to do its job more efficiently in every aspect, from sexual function to manual labor.

Goto Drinks In Times Of Health Distress:
I put 1 tablespoon of colloidal silver under my tongue at first sign of any cold, flu, unwell feeling.

Slowly sprinkle one capsule of Megahydrate and one of crystallized oxygen without herbs over a quart bottle of Whole foods Sparkling Mineral Water. You will have a health-giving drink that will make you feel better no matter what is wrong.

To one quart of pure water add ¾ teasp baking soda and 1 teaspoon of magnesium chloride. This makes magnesium bicarbonate, a tonic for the kidneys and the body.
(an internet search will easily guide you to these ingredients)

Chapter 20

> # *EVEN PEOPLE WHO HAVE BEEN "HEALTH CONSCIOUS" ALL THEIR LIVES BENEFIT FROM OXYGEN*

People who have been health conscious all their lives *especially* need oxygen! My mom believed that since dad had good insurance, all our medical needs should be attended to. She had come to be this way because she had watched her mother die needlessly due to lack of medical insurance.

After years of illness, it was discovered that because of my mom's prudently taking care of all our illnesses, I suffered from Chronic Systemic Candidiasis which caused me to be tired, suffering with mood swings, forgetfulness and confusion, prone to every infection that came around and basically miserable with a lot of little aches and pains caused by the candida, which is a parasitic yeast.

Thanks to the help of a medical sleuth, who discovered that I had chronic candidiasis, I am able to live a normal life again, because the multitude of doctors I was seeing had not a clue what was wrong with me. The candida had come from taking antibiotics all my life - - but after taking tetracycline for a year for acne and taking birth control pills, I became like a vegetable.

I was sick in the worst way, tired all the time and I knew I was dying. I tried many treatments, but taking oxygen (in the form of 10 drops of 3 percent food grade hydrogen peroxide in a glass of juice three times a day), along with a homeopathic preparation for candida has finally gotten the candida under control, winning a ten year, and probably a lifelong battle with candidiasis.

The disease has all kinds of symptoms, and, depending on the condition of a person's immune system, masks itself as multiple sclerosis, schizophrenia, autism, asthma, vaginal yeast infections, chemical sensitivity, arthritis and many others.

Some people who suffer with it simply get one yeast infection after another with no other apparent symptoms. However, I'll bet their mental functioning is affected as well.

If you suffer from too many yeast infections and the white tongue which is a telltale sign of candidiasis, sugar cravings (the candida, a parasite, makes you crave sugar so it can live), mood swings, backache, skin eruptions, lethargy, confusion and sore joints, you may be a victim of this harmless parasite which can go wild in the body if too many antibiotics or birth control pills disturb the body's natural balance.

Then it starts growing out of control, causing a whole host of symptoms that are often not associated with it. If antibiotics give you diarrhea, indigestion and respiratory problems, then you should strongly suspect candidiasis. If your doctor doesn't know about it, tell him so he can find out about it. Oxygen therapy, diet and exercise have helped many people to rid their bodies of this annoying pest.

I help people based on all I have learned fighting it. Most traditionally trained physicians don't know much about Systemic . Chronic Candidiasis. **The Well Mind Association Of Greater Washington**

Contact Alyce Ortuzar on 301.774.6617 for further information and to sign up for the newsletter.

If you want a homeopathic or naturopathic physician, contact the **National Center For Homeopathy**, 801 N. Fairfax, #306, Alexandria, Virginia 22314 or the **International Foundation For Homeopathy**, 2366 Eastlake Avenue, Seattle, Washington, 98105.

Or you may be able to do what thousands of others and I do: safely treat Candidiasis yourself by simply taking oxygen, taking the homeopathic remedy for Candida (which will cost you about four dollars and fifty cents), and following the diet in this book.

Exclude fruits for the first three months and exercise regularly. It is very important that you take pancreatic digestive enzymes to dissolve the toxins that have built up in your system. If the suggestions above do not cure you, they certainly will improve your condition. However, if your case is too severe, you may need to see a doctor.

Regular exercise is extremely important because it stimulates the immune system to activate killer cells that literally eat toxins like candida and other parasites and diseases. Eat garlic and take coenzyme Q_{10}.

I read that eating raw garlic massively killed candida and decided to try it as therapy. The problem was that every time I ate garlic, I could not stay awake.

When I questioned my doctor at that time, a holistic internist whose specialty is treating candidiasis, he told me that since the garlic killed massive amounts of candida when I ate it the toxins from the dead organisms in my blood were what made me so tired.

So I put forth a new effort to try eating garlic as therapy for my candidiasis. Another doctor had given me nystatin, an antifungal, but after five years at 80 dollars a month, it had not made that much of a difference.

One important question my doctor asked me was, "When was the last time you felt well?" I remembered that I had gotten a sinus infection a few years before and a series of other problems had followed it. At the time that I got the sinus infection and the doctor gave me antibiotics, I was so relieved, thinking, what would this infection have done if I had not gotten the antibiotics?

Well as it turned out, taking the antibiotics in the first place caused the problem. It was determined that the initial antibiotics that had been given for the sinus infection had pushed my chronic candidiasis into full bloom, leaving me tired and feeling frustrated and helpless because my vitality was gone.

Then my dermatologist prescribed 250 mg. of tetracycline twice a day for a year for my acne and at the end of that time, I was like a vegetable.

Candida impairs the immune system so that its victims are susceptible to every other opportunistic infection.

When I started eating massive amounts of garlic (one to three raw crushed cloves, depending on their size, in my food or salad everyday) for the first week I experienced the tiredness that I was told was from the dead candida in my blood.

After eating the garlic, I felt like heavy hands were pushing me down and even if I tried to exercise to oxygenate my blood, I simply did not have the strength. I had to give in, could not stay awake no matter where I was! But after eating garlic for a week, I was no longer sleepy. Not only was I not sleepy, I had lots more energy!

After about a month of eating garlic I noticed a change in my chronic candidiasis. Since garlic massively kills it, it was no longer as chronic, though it persisted.

There is a simple natural test that you can do to see if you have candida. Raw garlic massively kills it as well as many other parasitic organisms that invade the body. Take four or five of the globules that are attached to a garlic bulb. Mash the raw garlic with a fork and add to a raw salad. Lemon juice makes it delicious. If, after eating this raw garlic, you feel unnaturally tired, then there is a strong possibility that you have candida.

Taking oxygen will give you more relief from candida than anything I have seen. Eating raw garlic will help keep it under control. Just make sure you are not sensitive to raw garlic. If you develop a headache after eating garlic, make sure the garlic was fresh and that you did not eat too much. You can gradually increase your dosage. Vegetable enzymes and mineral water help.

The sleuth discovered it was my mom's fanatical quest to keep us healthy that caused me to get the candida in the first place. For every cold, every sore throat, she had us at the doctors where we were given medicines for colds, often antibiotics. *Since antibiotics only work on germs, because colds are caused by viruses, it does not make sense that anyone would take antibiotics for a cold.*

Yet every time our doctor gave me antibiotics, my cold seemed to get better. I discovered later that the cold was going to get better within a few days all by itself anyway, so the antibiotics were worthless and harmful.

Taking oxygen can maintain healthy oxygen levels to fight off aging and disease. The favored way to start is by squirting one spritz of a 3 percent solution of food grade hydrogen peroxide in juice once a day, preferably before bed in the beginning. Work up to twice a day, then three times. Take one hour before meals. The difference in vitality will be very noticeable.

Taking oxygen this way is absolutely safe, and will not interfere with medications or harm you in any way. Two weeks to a month after taking oxygen regularly you will notice an incredible new kind of clarity as it rids your body of pollutants that had been slowing you down in the past. The important thing to remember about oxygen is that it nourishes and helps the good bacteria and zaps anaerobic life, which is composed of harmful substances.

I had so many little health problems before I started to take oxygen. I had sore throats until I learned to gargle with food grade hydrogen peroxide. My gums stopped bleeding a few days after I started spraying my mouth with it before I brushed my teeth.

I keep a spray bottle of 3 percent food grade hydrogen peroxide to spray all raw foods. I prefer certified organically grown or as fresh and natural as I can get, but which does not mean that they could not have picked up environmental contaminants along the way. Since I don't know which ones were grown in manure, I soak all vegetables in one fourth cup of 3 percent food grade hydrogen peroxide in a pint of water for from five to fifteen minutes.

If you have an illness, you need to work up to three to five times a day if you start using oxygen this way, as I recommend you do. Spray your mouth once a day for three days, then twice a day for three days, then three times a day for three days. Doing this three or four times a day markedly increases the oxygenation of your body.

Modern practices of "refining" foods are responsible for a lot of modern chronic diseases, including tooth decay. *Food has powerful healing properties and should be eaten the way it comes from nature so our bodies can benefit from its medicinal properties. Continually ingesting processed and junk foods is one of the causes for the national health crisis in this country.*

Improper diet can seriously hamper health, especially when people ingest pollutants on a daily basis in their air and food as well. (Pollutants such as pesticides, herbicides, fertilizer, chemicals used in processing foods, car exhaust fumes and industrial contamination that get released into the air.) Taking oxygen is becoming widely known for helping reverse the harmful effects.

The following is reprinted with permission. © by Dr. Donsbach.

Miracle Oxygen

The recent explosion of interest in the oral and infusion use of hydrogen peroxide heralds one of the greatest advances in the treatment of ailments of mankind in recent history. The impact this will have on future generations is almost impossible to imagine. This simple substance, known for decades, has the ability to change the course of human suffering by releasing cleansing and purifying oxygen to the body.

All of my original research was done with hydrogen peroxide; all of the work done by the great Dr. Rosenow at Mayo Clinic and the work done at Baylor University used hydrogen peroxide. It is still the preferred intravenous infusion product and the one I will continue to use for external appli-

cations. For oral ingestion, however, I now believe the product of choice to be magnesium peroxide, and it may have even more to offer. The oxygen content is more stable than that in hydrogen peroxide and when it is chemically reduced, it leaves a very beneficial mineral, magnesium, as oxygen is released.

1. What we are really talking about, the substance that helps achieve the remarkable changes in the human body, is oxygen.

2. Magnesium peroxide is an excellent oxygen donor and the end result of its oral use is the same as hydrogen peroxide used orally.

Don't eat stale oil as it contains a large amount of harmful free radicals. Your nose will tell you which oils are stale.

Hydrogen Peroxide Facts

Kurt W. Donsbach, D.C., N.D., Ph.D.

There have been many incorrect statements regarding the ingestion of hydrogen peroxide and now, magnesium peroxide. I would like to address these so that you as a patient will not be misled and stop using a potentially beneficial product.

Myth #1: Any of the peroxides destroy friendly bacteria in the gut and require that you reintroduce fresh bacteria constantly if you are using the peroxide on a regular basis. The proof offered was that when you put hydrogen peroxide into a yogurt culture, the resultant yogurt was weak and watery.

FACTS: THE FRIENDLY BACTERIA IN THE GUT ARE AEROBIC, MEANING THEY LIVE AS AN OXYGEN-USING ORGANISM. If you want the opinion of the bible of bacteriology, check this out in *Bergey's Manual of Systematic Bacteriology* or *Clinical Diagnosis by Laboratory Methods* by Todd & Sanford. The addition of extra oxygen to the yogurt culture could have altered other factors in the milk used in the culture, rather than destroying the lactobacillus. The reference used by the writer was conspiciously lacking bacteria counts before and after the addition of the hydrogen peroxide! The truth is you help, not hinder, lactobacillus with H_2O_2

Myth #2: Oral ingestion of hydrogen peroxide promotes the growth of various viruses, including what has been called the EBV virus, the HIV virus and others.

FACTS: HYDROGEN PEROXIDE IS CAPABLE OF DESTROYING EACH AND EVERY ONE OF THESE VIRUSES IN LABORATORY TESTS. This does not necessarily mean that the same action occurs in the body, but it is a pretty good indicator. THE MOST IMPORTANT FACT REGARDING THIS ALLEGATION IS NOT WHETHER OR NOT HYDROGEN PEROXIDE KILLS OR STIMULATES A VIRUS, BUT HOW HYDROGEN PEROXIDE IS HANDLED BY THE BODY WHEN IT IS ABSORBED FROM THE GUT. What actually occurs is that the instant hydrogen peroxide crosses the intestinal barrier and enters the blood stream, the enzyme catalase splits the compound into water and free radical oxygen. This takes one molecule of catalase for every 10,000 molecules of hydrogen peroxide and uses up about 1/10,000 of a second. In approximately another 1/10,000 of a second you will see one free radical oxygen (O_1) join another free radical oxygen to form stable oxygen (O_2). Since this all takes approximately 1/5,000 of a second, when does the hydrogen peroxide have time to enter the circulatory channels and end up in the T cells where the HIV virus proliferates? Obviously it doesn't. THIS IS ALSO THE ANSWER TO THE CLAIM THAT FREE RADICAL OXYGEN WILL CAUSE CELLULAR DAMAGE. THE FREE RADICAL OXYGEN HAS AN EXTREMELY SHORT LIFE IN THE BLOOD STREAM ONLY AND NEVER GETS CLOSE TO CELLS!

© By Dr. Kurt W. Donsbach. Reprinted with permission.

Before you start taking oxygen, notice the symptoms you have, and how you are feeling. It is helpful to sit back, take an evaluation and write down all the physical symptoms you are having. They might be as slight as "minor stiffness in left knee upon arising that goes away as the day passes, headaches from time to time, stomachache after eating onions."

You could even narrow it down by noting on your calendar when each headache occurs to see if there is some pattern of regularity. You may begin to notice that your headaches occur after eating certain foods.

Eating eggs makes some people who are allergic to them irritable. Monitor how your symptoms change with oxygen therapy, and your improvement. Not one person who went on oxygen therapy reported any negative response.

One of the reasons for the increase in asthma is our polluted air. A 1993 study of six large cities showed that even in areas that meet Federal air quality standards, the air can shorten life, blaming the smallest particles like auto exhaust as most harmful. Everyday when you walk out your door you walk through a field of invisible toxins in the air.

If you have asthma, taking oxygen and vitamin C may be two of the most important things you ever do in your life. If your asthma seems to be getting worse not better, you may need one of the new inhalers that help greatly during an asthma attack. Make sure your home is free of dust mites. See a homeopathic doctor.

Rise In Asthma Deaths Is Tied
To Ignorance Of Many Physicians

"The death rate from asthma has more than doubled since 1978 in the United States. And worried officials of the National Institutes of Health attribute the trend in part to the lack of education and training of the primary-care doctors who treat the overwhelming majority of asthmatics."[81]

---

[81]   © 1993 by The New York Times, New York, NY by Lawrence K. Altman, M.D.

Whichever form of oxygen you start with, proceed with responsibility. If hesitant about taking it as we have been discussing; I recommend you start with Cherry Berry Oxy Toddy, to get used to the taste, and after taking it in that form for a month or so, you may want to take it in a less expensive form, or try the crystal oxygen pills.

Many people start by taking one dose of Oxy Toddy (there are ten drops in a dose or half an ounce) every night before bed for a week. The following week they take two doses a day. Many people work up to three doses, which is thought to be ideal for healthy individuals.

Oxygen can be taken four or five times a day during an illness, then drop back to two or three times a day. Make sure you get at least six glasses of water or liquids everyday. Some find it beneficial to increase their dosage to 20 drops of oxygen per dose if it can be tolerated. Listen to your body and let it be the judge.

If you choose to take the crystal oxygen pills, here's a word of caution: they impart a super amount of energy and greatly increase libido! They are a superior product and if one is too much for you, cut a capsule in half and take one half, one fourth or one eighth for each dose. It is best taken with a full glass of water during the day and never before bed. Monitor the effect the crystal oxygen has on you. It stimulates me so much I break one capsule into eight. Empty gel caps can be found at health food stores.

I have read that some people say that when they first started taking oxygen they got a nauseous feeling, but my mother, sisters and I, nor any of the people I know who take it did not. The reason for the nausea is the same as the reason garlic makes people with chronic candidiasis sleepy and weighed down; *correct amounts of oxygen or garlic massively kill toxins in the body*, and candida is one of them, therefore the toxins from the dead organisms in the blood cause tiredness. While you rest, your immune system gets rid of them. Before long, they're all gone and you have all this new vitality!

Chapter 21

> ### FIGHTING CANCER AND AIDS WITH OXYGEN, HOMEOPATHY, AND MINERALS, A CURE IN MOST CASES

At this moment an inexpensive form of oxygen is being used in Germany to treat people who have full blown AIDS to fully recover. I think any measure that cures AIDS or cancer, especially one that <u>works</u>, that is natural and does no harm, should be used. Many patients report that they have had incredible healings using a natural mineral, Colloidal Silver. According to Living Energy Systems on the www, "It is impossible for sincle-celled germs to mutate into silver-resistant forms, as happens with conventional antibiotics. Therefore, no tolerance to colloidal silver ever develops. Also, colloidal silver cannot interact or interfere with other medicine being taken. Inside the body, colloidal silver forms no toxic compounds nor reacts with anthing other than pathogens. It is a truly safe, natural remedy and a great alternative to conventional treatments." Every disease condition improved drastically with its use. I predict it will be a treatment that revolutionizes healing in the future.

With oxygen therapy, people with AIDS not only fully recovered, they really did return to being HIV-. The same is true for 75% of the "untreatable" cancer patients that go to Hospital Santa Monica (1-800-359-6547). This therapy is done under very safe, controlled conditions and none of the patients have experienced ill effects from it. The therapy is most effective during the early stages of cancer and AIDS.

An article in Medical Hypotheses[82] by H. C. Greenspan about the role of reactive oxygen in AIDS stresses that oxidative stress is one important reason HIV progresses.

In another article in the September 1993 issue of the Journal of Clinical Gastroenterology[83] entitled **Does Ozone Alleviate AIDS Diarrhea?** three gentlemen, Carpendale, Freeberg and Griffiss, all M.D.'s, discovered that intractable AIDS diarrhea could be cured with daily infusions of oxygen in the form of ozone. They found that one person remained free of all symptoms of disease and concluded that ozone, being safe and effective, should be used.

Further discussions noted that if ozone could infiltrate the parenchyma of the liver to inactivate hepatitis, there was no reason why it could not inactivate HIV or any other virus from the walls of the colon.

Ozone has also been used successfully to treat bacterial, protozoal, viral diseases including hepatitis (B), herpes and zosters. Only recently has it been discovered to inactivate HIV. It also produces interferon in blood. When it is injected into withdrawn blood it inactivates the virus. When the blood is reinjected into the AIDS patient, the dead viruses act as a vaccine and cause the person's body to make antibodies to HIV.

If you have AIDS there are three different methods of taking and using oxygen that have been effective in eliminating it. Not all AIDS cases respond to oxygen therapy, but in studies, it succeeded more than it failed. Any success is better than what other sources are getting, which is none.

No one has been successful at treating end-stage AIDS. Whatever stage you are in, your hope and positive feelings are among the best weapons you can use

[82]   © 1993 Medical Hypotheses (40,85-92) Longman Group UK Ltd.

[83]   © 1993 by Raven Press, Ltd. New York. From the Rehabilitation Medicine Service, San Francisco Veterans Administration Medical Center (SFVAMC) and the Department of Orthopaedic Surgery, University of California, San Francisco School of Medicine (MTC.,JMG) San Francisco, CA, USA.

to fight it along with the proper fuel for your body to strengthen it and the proper therapy for you. Below are the three ways that have been effective in completely eliminating AIDS with oxygen:

- By mouth. Three percent (preferably food grade) hydrogen peroxide either squirted into the mouth or into a glass of juice (the equivalent of 10 drops). If squirted into the mouth, swish around, especially between the teeth, allow to foam and spit out. The atoms of hydrogen drop off and pure O_2 is absorbed through the mouth and throat. This method has not been successful for everyone, but it has been most successful when implemented in the early stages and supplemented with vitamins and minerals and a proper diet. Exercise, if possible, is also helpful.

- By removing blood from the patient, infusing it with a special hydrogen peroxide or ozone and returning to the patient. This method is moderately successful.

- By infusing correct amounts of ozone into the rectum and/or ear. Successful in many cases after the correct dosage is determined.

To locate a physician who can give you oxidative therapy, call or write The International Bio-Oxidative Medicine Foundation, PO Box 891-154, Oklahoma City, OK 73113-1205, phone number 405-478-IBOM (4266) or 1-800-235-4788. There is a small fee for the list of doctors. If you are a physician, they have training in administering oxidative therapy.

Shouldn't any safe, natural method of effectively combatting AIDS be applied? Right now we need to get busy and change the legislation that says it is illegal to use oxygen therapy to cure AIDS.

A good source of information on oxygen therapies is:
Well Mind Association Of Greater Washington
Contact Alyce Ortuzar on 301.774.6617 for further information and to sign up for the newsletter.

In some cases, when infused into the blood in correct proportions, oxygen can arrest many forms of cancer and AIDS if it is used in the early stages. It sometimes works in the latter stages. Contact Hospital Santa Monica, 619-428-1146, or 1-800-359-6547 for cancer treatment. They are especially good for hopeless cases and terminal illnesses.

Following is a testimonial from a person who completely cured himself of full-blown AIDS by taking oxygen by mouth (as I did) and other supplements. You can contact him by phone or mail if you would like to confirm his cure. He had been traveling around the country trying to increase awareness about oxygen therapy for curing AIDS by speaking to groups and organizations, but is now home again. Please call after 6 pm and do not ask him to call you back as I don't want him to have to return a million phone calls.

There are testimonials from people who have had complete cure and remission of cancer and other diseases simply from taking an inexpensive form of oxygen. Jim and I are two of them.

If you are HIV+ and have no symptoms of disease and don't or can't afford oxygen therapy (which is very affordable) you may be able to use inexpensive, effective oral oxygen therapy. Ten drops of 3 percent hydrogen peroxide in a glass of juice three times a day, micronutrient supplementation, diet, exercise and homeopathic medicines to delay the onset of the disease indefinitely, and possibly, return you to   HIV-. Phytochemicals, the healing substances found in fruits and vegetables, Coenzyme Q_{10}, enzymes, peptides, flavonoids, phenolic compounds like vitamin E have hold promise in the treatment of AIDS.[84]

If I were HIV+ I would get the physician-administered oxygen therapy to make me negative and not wait for the disease to strike.

---

[84]   © 1993 Medical Hypotheses (40,85-92) Longman Group UK Ltd. pg. 90.

*Jim McPherson * 219 E. Thompson Street * Philadelphia, PA 19125 * (215) 425 - 0056*

April 30, 1993

Following is a true and accurate account of my personal experience with AIDS and the course I chose to pursue in its treatment. This information is being shared not to suggest that this regimen will work for everyone but in hope that others may know that there are alternatives to the traditional and largely unsuccessful protocols and modalities of treatment. AIDS does not have to be a death sentence.

Having always been an extremely energetic person all throughout my life, I found it quite unusual that during the summer months of 1992 I was continually feeling drained and weak. After just beginning a new job with a major national publication, I was tested and found to be HIV+. My initial medical tests to determine the extent of the illness showed that my CD4 count was at 72, classifying me as having full-blown AIDS. This was in early September, 1992.

Within about three to four weeks of my initial testing, I began to experience symptoms of the advancement of the disease including; severe night sweats, a continuous fever of 102+, constant and frequent diarrhea, difficulty in keeping food down, a general loss of appetite and an extreme weakness in my legs which was often accompanied by difficulty in walking. I also began to develop what appeared to be water blisters on various parts of my body, especially my hands and feet. I had also lost approximately 14 pounds within a 3 1/2 week period.

Already a believer of the benefits of natural products and their benefits to the human body, I had been taking a cold processed whole-leaf Aloe Vera concentrate (1,200 mg/day of the Active Ingredients) from Aloe Nique' and R PUR Aloe and a potassium mineral supplement manufactured by Matol Botanical, International called Km (2 1/2 ounces/day) which is formulated from 14 different botanicals. In addition to these, I began to take a combination of herbal extracts from Pure Herbs, Ltd. including myrrh (60 drops/day), hyssop (40 drops/day), broad beans (40 drops/day) and a formulation called B.P. - W containing bee pollen, buckthorn, greasewood, inkberry, peach leaf, prickly ash, red clover, and stillingia (60 drops/day). I also began an intake of bovine colostrum whey processed by Sterling Technology (1 ounce/day), a 35% food grade hydrogen peroxide solution (9-75 drops/day) and a brown powder affectionately known as "Pygmy Dirt." This course of nutritional supplementation began approximately the second week of October.

The next series of diagnostic testing was done during the first week of November. Those results brought back the following positive information. When initially diagnosed by the American Red Cross as HIV+ in early September, it was also confirmed that I tested positive for Hepatitis B. The November test results showed no sign of the Hepatitis B surface antigen. Even more encouraging was the fact that these early November test results showed a CD4 count of 810.

Physically, I felt much better than I had previously, with a lot of my strength and endurance returning. I still had some mild symptoms of night sweats and an occasional fever. The weakness in my legs and the difficulty in walking disappeared altogether. The blisters had almost totally dissipated and I began to gain much of my weight back.

I continued with my herbal and nutritional supplementation and received my next series of diagnostic testing the second week of December with the good news that all my blood counts were within acceptable range and a CD4 count of 1092. By this time, physically I was feeling extremely well and almost back to the healthy, energetic level to which I had been accustomed most of my life. Emotionally and psychologically, I was pulled between the return of my physical health and the loss of my job due to my illness and the resulting severe financial pressure being placed on my life.

However, just after the previous series of tests were run in early December, one element of my treatment changed with some highly noticeable side effects. Everything remained the same except that I was no longer including the bovine colostrum in my therapy. Within about two and a half weeks after discontinuing the colostrum, I began to experience severe and frequent stomach pains which accompanied a painful belching. In addition, I began to run a moderate fever which remained fairly constant and the return of the constant diarrhea. When tested again on the 19th of January, 1993, my diagnostics showed a great reduction in my lymphocytes, significant increase in my polys (indicating that my body was involved in combating an infection) and more significantly, a decrease in my CD4 count to 702.

Perhaps it is through the network of others who hear about my experiences that hope can be spread. I also continue to search for the successful experiences that others have to share with regards to their particular naturopathic and alternative therapies. I sincerely believe that there are many answers to this disease and many alternative regimens which will work. I cannot say that the course I have chosen is the answer for everyone and I invite others to contact me, either to hear of my regimen or to tell me of theirs. I know that it is only through many of us working together that we can effectively win this war.

I am also attempting to develop and organize a non-profit buyers' service for those who wish to follow an alternative therapy regimen but simply cannot afford its components. Unfortunately, the majority of those who are in need of the alternative therapies and naturopathic supplementation are those to whom they are financially unavailable. Through this buyers' service, I hope to make these alternative and naturopathic supplementation therapies available to anyone, regardless of financial capability.

I have come to understand that this is so much more than simply a physical disease; that there are also many very important spiritual, sociological and psychological implications at play as well. Not everyone will be victorious in their battle against AIDS but I want to do my part to help those who truly do want to win and are willing to survive. Perhaps by sharing my experiences, I am helping to make a difference in the lives of others. I openly ask the assistance of anyone who has the capacity or desire to assist me in helping others. I cannot do it alone. But perhaps with the caring and the sharing efforts of others, we can make a world of difference.

I welcome anyone who wishes to receive more information to call upon me as I will be delighted to share my experiences in greater detail as well as to assist in locating sources of the individual components of my own and other nutritional supplementation regimens. I highly caution anyone who wishes to pursue this or any other naturopathic or supplementation therapy to be certain of the purity and strength of your supplementation simply because your life may very well depend upon it. I have spent a lot of time and effort searching for the purest and highest quality supplements and can provide source information to anyone who requests it. Afterall, I know that many others feel as I do; that when dealing with your health, the quality and purity of the products you use are of utmost importance.

I am always open to new ideas and thoughts and I welcome input from anyone who hears of my quest and am truly thankful for the opportunity to share my experiences with others. I hope that the above information is of value to you or someone you love or care for. I sincerely hope that I can be of assistance in helping others to avoid unnecessary pain and loss so frequently associated with AIDS and HIV.
I offer my blessings of hope - and health - and happiness.
Sincerely,

Jim McPherson

Jim McPherson

I recently heard a news report which stated that some Italian researchers have found that some individuals, depending on their immune systems, can get AIDS from kissing. How do I know if I'm one of them or not? To make kissing safe I spray my mouth and the mouth of the person I'm kissing with 3 percent hydrogen peroxide solution before and after kissing. Sounds a little silly, doesn't it? But this solution will also protect you from herpes.[85] I don't mean go out and kiss someone with herpes everyday. I recommend you don't kiss anyone with herpes!

Speaking of kissing, some of the things we need to protect ourselves from during oral sex are AIDS, herpes, staph and strep infections and a number of others. Use the hydrogen peroxide rule for kissing and for oral sex with an uninfected partner also.

It is a small measure of protection that could be the difference between life and death. If you are sure that the person you are having sex with is clean (uninfected with anything), and insist on having sex without a condom, a light film of 3 percent solution should be sprayed on the hands and rubbed on the penis before having sex anyway.

It should be used each time you have sex along with a germicidal spermicide inserted into the vagina. To doubly protect yourself and kill germs and sperm, insert spermicide inside the condom and in the vagina.

A heavy film will cause burning. A light film will mix and be diluted by body fluids, spermicide and vaginal lubricant. It may take a few tries before you get the right dosage to prevent stinging. Douche immediately afterwards with three tablespoons of 3 percent hydrogen peroxide in 8 oz. of water.

---

[85]   I kissed someone with active herpes, doused my mouth with peroxide and 15 years have passed and I have never come down with herpes once. I also helped several people who were experiencing their first herpes lesion on the lip who have remained herpes free to this day. One of them was 17 years ago. If a cotton ball soaked in a 3% solution of hydrogen peroxide is taped to the first herpes eruption (and this works only if the first eruption is on the lips, since I have not treated it otherwise) and allowed to remain there for several hours, the ideal time is during sleep, then the peroxide will suck out every drop of the herpes virus from your body. It will not recur. Make sure the cotton ball is soaked enough to continuously feed hydrogen peroxide to the entire herpes lesion.

Next night it is okay to insert an acidophilus capsule deep up into the vagina just before bed to restore the natural flora of the vagina. Taking acidophilus orally can restore it also.

People have advised me not to recommend any measures for people who have sex without a condom. I am not recommending that anyone not use a condom. I am directing this information to people who insist on living dangerously and proceeding without.

I don't think they should die if they choose to go without either. The above measures should be used each time you have sex along with a germicidal spermicide inserted into the vagina. An excellent one is the French, product, **Taro Cap**. There are some suitable American ones also, although they do not compare to the French one. Nonoxyl 9, the ingredient used in most American made spermicide, is also an antiseptic, but do not rely on it alone.

I would never have sex without a condom unless I was with a longtime sex partner and we knew we were both monogamous and HIV- (by this I mean since we both tested for HIV 2-3 months previously and have both been monogamous since). Even then, I would coat his penis with a light film of 3 percent hydrogen peroxide. Even when using a condom, it is recommended that you use a light film of 3 percent hydrogen peroxide on the hands and full strength in the mouth during and after oral sex with an uninfected partner (and definitely with someone you don't know about, which you should not be having unprotected sex with).

At the time of conception, even though the fetus is enclosed in a sac, germs and bacteria should be kept out of the vagina because next to deficiency in the mother, they are a major cause of birth defects.

Having sex during pregnancy presents a tremendous risk of introducing bacteria into the vagina at this critical time. This is when you should be at your hygienic best.

> ## What Are The Guidelines For Not Getting AIDS?

Trying to get any of the agencies in Washington to give the guidelines for AIDS is not easy. No one wants to be responsible for being the one who said something that turned out to be untrue. Therefore, they say nothing. The most recent literature I found was dated 1988, issued when Everett Koop was Surgeon General. The guidelines are listed as risky behavior:

Sharing drug needles and syringes

Anal sex, with or without a condom

Vaginal or oral sex with someone who shoots
drugs or engages in anal sex

Sex with someone you don't know well
(a pickup or prostitute) or with
someone you know has several sex partners

Unprotected sex (without a condom)
with an infected person

Any exchange of infected blood,
semen or vaginal fluids can spread
the virus and put you at great risk

So, after reading that list, and the next two headlines, I see how it could be possible for some people to be able to contract AIDS from kissing. Certainly it could be contracted through an open sore or cavity in the mouth if you kissed an infected person.

But I spoke to at least ten doctors who say you cannot get AIDS from kissing, except through a sore in the mouth or cavity. But suppose you were involved with someone and you loved kissing him or her. If you spent an hour kissing him in a whole evening, haven't you traded enough saliva to get almost anything contagious the other person has?

You can get AIDS from oral sex, yet I remember reading in the news a few years ago that AIDS could not be transmitted by oral sex. How many people got AIDS because they missed the retraction of that statement? It seems logical to me that if you can get AIDS from oral sex you could get it from kissing.

To test yourself for AIDS, most local health departments provide testing free or for a 5 or 10 dollar administrative fee. They use a number rather than a name system to protect your anonymity.

Theory Links AIDS To Malaria
Experiments

"Dr. Charles Gilks of Oxford University and the Kenya Medical Research Institute has discovered reports of a series of little-known malaria experiments in which people were inoculated with fresh blood from monkeys and chimpanzees. He suggests that this blood may have infected humans with primate viruses that were the ancestors of the AIDS virus."[86]

Today there is a widespread view that the overuse of antibiotics in our culture precipitated and perpetuates AIDS, our modern dreaded disease. It is speculated that several deadly diseases like drug-resistant TB and drug-resistant gonorrhea have come about because of the incorrect use and abuse of antibiotics. We use hundreds of thousands of tons of antibiotics on crops and in animal feed.

These strong drugs, when taken repeatedly, greatly compromise the human immune system and impair the organism's future abilities to fight disease. Antibiotics and cortisone are also immunosuppressants and thus, increase the chances of getting anything. On the other hand, there are homeopathic medicines that cure bacterial and viral infections and stimulate the immune system to be stronger in the same process.

When these weakened humans come in contact with what has come to be the AIDS virus, they are more susceptible to it than individuals with uncompromised immune systems.

There are stories that AIDS originated in Africa from the practice of using one needle to inject many patients. Antibiotics are available over the counter in Haiti, where there is also a high incidence of AIDS.

What we have discovered is that people with weakened immune systems, poor nutrition and repeated incidences of infections with the use of broad-spectrum antibiotics to cure them are at greater risk of catching anything, and especially AIDS.

---

[86]   © 1991 by The New York Times Company. By Gina Kolata. Reprinted by permission.

Some have said repeatedly that the use of a live smallpox vaccine in Africa years ago may have triggered a dormant AIDS virus.

Although there has been much speculation on the subject, I believe the AIDS virus can live out of the body and go into a dormant state as so many bacteria and viruses can and then reactivate itself after it finds a warm, moist host.

Please read on to see what homeopathic authorities have to say about treating AIDS:

"It is common for homeopaths to report that patients with AIDS or ARC seem to experience reduced recurrence and intensity of infection. Individual homeopaths also report that people who are HIV+ do not develop AIDS or ARC very often. London homeopaths Michael Strange, Tina Head, and Melissa Assilem, whose Lavender Hill Homeopathic Centre specializes in gay health, report to having treated several hundred HIV+ patients. They estimate that 90 percent of their HIV+ patients have not yet developed AIDS."

Reprinted with permission of Dana Ullman, from **Discovering Homeopathy**, published by North Atlantic Books, Berkeley CA. 1991, pg. 229.

"Many PWAs get fungal infections. Los Angeles homeopath and acupuncturist Janet Zand has found the following medicines to be helpful in treating these conditions: *Thuja, Sulphur*, and various homeopathic nosodes (a nosode is a medicine potentized from a pathogenic tissue)."

Reprinted with permission of Dana Ullman, from **Discovering Homeopathy**, published by North Atlantic Books, Berkeley CA. 1991, pg. 230.

"San Francisco homeopath Dr. Laurence Badgley reported on a six month study of 36 of his patients with AIDS, ARC or HIV+ treated with homeopathy and other natural therapies. He observed an average 13 percent increase in T4 helper cells and an average increase of two pound weight. He has found the following medicines to be particularly helpful in the homeopathic treatment of people with AIDS: *Typhoidinum* (typhoid nosode) *Badiagia* (fresh water sponge), Cyclosporin."

Reprinted with permission of Dana Ullman, from **Discovering Homeopathy**, published by North Atlantic Books, Berkeley CA. 1991, pg. 231.

"Homeopath Michael Strange has observed that his patients who get Pneumocystis carninii pneumonia (PCP) nonetheless get less severe bouts of it. He notes some of the common medicines he has used successfully in treating the acute episodes of PCP are *Bryonia* (wild hops) *China* (Cinchona bark), *Pulsatilla* (windflower) *Silica*.

Strange has also noted that homeopathic medicines seem to slow or stop new Karposi's sarcoma (KS) lesions. The medicines he has used successfully include *Phosphorus*, *Lachesis* and *Crotalus horridus*. Strange has also potentized doses of cytotoxic drugs *(Vinblastin 12, Vincristin 12, Bleomycin 6)* in patients who were prescribed conventional doses of them for their KS lesions in the lungs. In the two cases in which Strange has prescribed these homeopathic doses of cytotoxic drugs he has managed to avert all side effects of the conventional drugs without interfering with the effectiveness of the treatment."

Reprinted with permission of Dana Ullman, from **Discovering Homeopathy**, published by North Atlantic Books, Berkeley CA. 1991, pg. 230.

"London homeopath Michael Strange reports having approximately 50 people with AIDS under his care. Only five of these 50 people died during 1990, and the majority of his patients with AIDS are fit and active.

Although these results do not sound miraculous, they are actually quite significant considering the serious and progressive nature of AIDS."

Reprinted with permission of Dana Ullman, from **Discovering Homeopathy**, published by North Atlantic Books, Berkeley CA. 1991, pg. 231.

"Greek physician Spiro Diamantidis, who chairs the homeopathic commission for the Greek Ministry of Health and Welfare, recently reported on the treatment of 12 HIV+ patients, three of whom have AIDS, and four of whom had ARC, and five of whom were HIV+ with swollen lymph glands. These patients utilized homeopathic medicines solely, and each showed complete remission of symptoms and normalization of immune panels."

Reprinted with permission of Dana Ullman, from **Discovering Homeopathy**, published by North Atlantic Books, Berkeley CA. 1991, pg. 232.

"Some of the common medicines that Strange has found to be helpful are *Arsenicum* (arsenic), *Phosphorus, Natrum mur* (salt), *Pulsatilla* (windflower), *Sepia* (cuttlefish), *Tuberculinum* (tuberculosis nosode), *Medorrhinum* (gonorrhea nosode), and *Carcinosin* (cancer nosode).

Belgian homeopaths Drs. Maurice Jenaer and Bernard Marichal have recently reported on a trial conducted in Africa utilizing a combination of homeopathic medicines. In a preliminary test using 28 people with AIDS (14 men and 14 women), they observed statistically significant improvement in people with AIDS from homeopathically potentized doses of *RNA, DNA, Cyclosporin* and a rabbit antibody called *Polypeptide Anti-Atypies.*

This study showed that those patients treated with homeopathic medicines... had one-half as many infections, and one-sixth as many bouts of diarrhea. The untreated patients lost an average of 22 pounds, while the treated patients actually gained 3 pounds."

Reprinted with permission of Dana Ullman, from **Discovering Homeopathy**, published by North Atlantic Books, Berkeley CA. 1991. pg. 232.

Some homeopaths have found value in *Thuja* (tree of life), Syphilinum (syphilis nosode), various *Mercury* preparations, various *Calcarea* (calcium) preparations, *Sulphur, Lycopodium* (club moss), *Crotalus horridus* (rattlesnake), *Conium* (hemlock), and *Bromium.*

Reprinted with permission of Dana Ullman, from **Discovering Homeopathy**, published by North Atlantic Books, Berkeley CA. 1991, pg. 232.

Recent research has shown that hypericin, a compound within the homeopathic medicine *Hypericum*, inhibits retroviruses in vitro and in vivo. A 1989 survey reported that 80-90 percent of 24 AIDS patients who used it experienced some benefit. This survey also discovered that liver enzymes improved in almost every case. Though not a homeopathic dose, 60-90 drops of the tincture three times a day, or 70 mg. of hypericin seem therapeutic. No side effects have been reported at these doses.

Reprinted with permission of Dana Ullman, from **Discovering Homeopathy,** published by North Atlantic Books, Berkeley CA. 1991. pg. 232.

In my personal discussions with homeopathic practitioners, I have learned that little progress with homeopathic medicines can be expected in the treatment of people with end-stage AIDS or with PWAs with neurological involvement. The best results come from those who are HIV+ without serious immunological problems, those with ARC, those recently diagnosed with AIDS, and patients who avoid conventional drugs. Several homeopaths have observed that progress from homeopathic medicines diminishes if the person concurrently utilizes certain powerful conventional medical treatments, specifically AZT, or if they recurrently take antibiotics. However, now that physicians are recommending lower doses of AZT, homeopaths are observing that homeopathic medicines are more able to act effectively.

Reprinted with permission of Dana Ullman, from **Discovering Homeopathy,** published by North Atlantic Books, Berkeley CA. 1991, pg. 233.

According to Ed McCabe in his paper **Successful AIDS Treatments** (available through **The Family News** 1-800-284-6263 for 5 dollars) six doctors have removed all disease markers and viruses from over 300 AIDS patients and returned them to HIV- using oxygen therapy. His book entitled **Oxygen Therapies** is very relevant. Following are some excerpts from the paper:

AN ABBREVIATED LIST OF
IMPORTANT MEDICAL OZONE EVENTS AND
REFERENCES IN CHRONOLOGICAL ORDER
WITH A CONCENTRATION ON

SUCCESSFUL AIDS TREATMENTS

SIX INDEPENDENT DOCTORS HAVE REMOVED
ALL DISEASE MARKERS AND VIRUSES FROM OVER
300 AIDS PATIENTS AND RETURNED THEM TO

HIV NEGATIVE

BY ED McCABE
AUTHOR OF
"OXYGEN THERAPIES"

COPYRIGHT 1991, 1992
BY ED McCABE

Barron's goes on to talk of the cost and effectiveness of currently approved therapies. "The Department of Health And Human Services states the cost of care this year for HIV positive patients is $5.8 billion, and will double in two years." and, "available treatments have only marginally extended the lives of most patients, and some of the more effective drugs are marred by significant toxicities of their own... AZT is highly toxic... FDA approved DDI October 1991. DDI's side effects 'occasionally fatal' pancreatitis, peripheral neuropathy... sometimes the patient can't walk." and, "solutions are years away ... up to 25 years away."

Here's where the statistics get interesting. Barron's continues: Tax supported NIH - National Institute of Health's AIDS research budget rises to 851 million dollars, up from zero 10 years ago. As of August 1991, the manufacturer of AZT took in $315 million dollars on sales of it.

1992 Jan   Recently fired Center For Disease Control employee appears on the news and says he was fired for telling the truth, so now he will tell all he knows. He states that the real figures are that 57 million people have the AIDS virus.

January 1992 Captain Michael Shannon, Deputy Surgeon General for the Canadian Naval Forces has 350 scientists under him. He is negotiating with Medizone to commence a 2 1/2 million dollar ozone medical research study that will include blood sterilization, animal trials, and more. The Canadian Government realized that if a major event occurs, their armed forces' blood supply would be inadequate in its present condition.

April 1992 I interviewed Dr. Eric Satori MD, and one of his 50 "best case" former AIDS patients, Mr. John Burdick. Dr. Satori told me the results he was getting with his own brand of direct IV ozone therapy which also includes mental conditioning: "To remove the reason the patient gets diseased." So far, he had 149 AIDS patients become healthy, 50 of which sero-converted to negative and became virus free by combining ozone with special vitamin, peroxide, mineral, thymus, and homeopathic supplements. He reports he commonly got results in only 12 days because he has been improving therapy daily during 10 years of clinical fine tuning. His ozone dosage protocol depended upon body size, but an 185 pound man might be injected with 18 to 20 35cc. syringes of 70 mcg/ml ozone per day. He states it is important, in order to kill the viruses, to give the full dosages right at first to the patient, before the body turns on the alternate pathways to deactivate the ozone.

June 1992 Dr. John Pittman, Raleigh, NC started using ozone autohemotherapy combined with detoxification and dietary and nutritional supplementation therapy since 1991. He is now using direct IV ozone infusions. "Typically seeing dramatic results. Clinically significant improvements in well being, patients were gaining weight, any opportunistic infections they had cleared right up, including diarrhea and thrush. The people who have been on AZT, I just do not ever see big turnarounds in their T cell counts. That fits, because they blasted their bone marrow with it, and there's not much to rebuild there. Even clinically though they look great with the ozone. The patients that never took AZT, there's a definite turnaround in their T cell counts with the combination therapy." In June of 1992, the head of the AIDS clinical study group at Duke University attacked Dr. Pittman's successful work in a local newspaper. He said "Using ozone is totally bizarre, I've never heard of anything like it before in my life," and without any inquiry, reported Dr. Pittman to the state medical board. The same scenario and excuses were also acted out against Dr. Pittman by a local self proclaimed AIDS activist. The ensuing political pressure forced Dr. Pittman to temporarily abandon his successful research, although a high level of interest was generated in the use of ozone among top state officials.

June 1992 Two months earlier, in April, ozone doctor Eric Satori M.D. was arrested and jailed under a trumped up charge. In June he was home in Fort Washington, Maryland and saw a large plain black "government type" car heading for his house. He ran out the back, hid in the woods, and 4 plainclothes agents tore the house apart, pulling pictures off the wall, emptying drawers and throwing everything onto the floor. Then they left. No notice was left behind explaining who they were or what authority was exercised. Dr. Satori, fearing for his

Unless humanity as a whole - and it just might emerge from the direction of the littlest of the "little guys" - finally wakes up and decides to collectively let ozone out of the bag, then there might be only widespread sickness and death in every family. Their sins of letting others take responsibility for their own lives will come to visit and live with them. Then where will they drive their shiny new car every day? Why, to the AIDS ward and the cemetery.

PRESENT Thousands of German, Swiss, and other European MD's are getting rid of AIDS and many other diseases in thousands of patients with continuing use of various ozone therapies.

In the US, the ozone medical treatments remain rumors not fully explained in the media. Because the media often erroneously does the public a disservice by interchanging the word "smog" with the word "ozone," one LA man was admitted to a hospital due to poisoning. TV says smog is "ozone," and he heard in the underground that ozone cured AIDS, so he started chasing busses exhausting what he thought was ozone, and deeply breathing the bus fumes in a desperate, yet tragically misguided attempt to cure himself. Smog is tons of hydrogen, nitrogen, carbon and sulphur. The ozone in smog is so tiny an amount that it's measured in only parts per million. This fact is ignored on the nightly news. Medical ozone is none of this, it is always only 100% energized pure oxygen, a whole different animal. Almost zero side effects have surfaced in all the millions of medical ozone treatments given. Almost every disease responds favorably when a wholistic approach is taken during the course of medical ozone treatment. The most common side effects reported are increased energy, an increased sense of well being, and clearer thinking. Over 5,000 medical ozone machines have been sold in Europe and are presently in use by as many doctors.

SUMMARY

For now, the oxygen wars continue unabated. The shameful politics and non-responses of our medical system are so bad that even the most unaware are hard pressed to believe we are simply facing a whole bunch of coincidental ignorance and errors. Government, media and medical bigwigs as a whole continue to strangely ignore or disparage the over fifty years history of millions of applications of safe, non-toxic ozone therapy, and, in fact, continue to actively use S.W.A.T. teams, the FDA, the DEA, the IRS, and jail terms to suppress any further medical ozone research. People suffer tragically and die needlessly, while many who love their families have their hearts slowly broken watching their significant others waste away. Rumors circulate on national talk shows about planned genocide.

Due to outright hostility, suppression, or at least non-response by our authorities, desperate people who are facing no alternative to their eventual death from AIDS, cancer or other killers are being forced into the unregulated "ozone underground." In any medical underground, where a therapy is not officially sanctioned or publicly known, mixed in along with a few shining humanitarians will always be con artists, scams, repression, and yellow journalism. You and your family deserve better than this.

As we saw, the U.S. Office Of Technology Assessment says that 95% of all the drugs on the market have not been proven to work. Keeping this statistic in mind, does this mean that since ozone has been proven to work well on the international scene for over 50 years, then medical ozone is therefore proven more effective than 95% of our commonly used "approved" remedies?

There are approved drugs for AIDS, AZT and DDI. AZT is "highly toxic" according to the newspapers, and DDI is being given to AIDS patients even though they never finished testing it. In light of the extreme threat to the public health from AIDS - perhaps up to 40+ million people scheduled to die as of today, perhaps including you or a loved one - and in light of all these doctors reporting patients coming up safely HIV negative due to medical ozone, don't you think ozone therapy should be immediately investigated, announced on the

When taken in the early stages of AIDS and cancer, oxygen along with vitamin and mineral supplementation, proper diet and exercise have been an effective cure for AIDS in over 300 documented cases. A person's overall health is an important factor in obtaining a cure. Oxygen can be used as a health preserver because it nourishes and strengthens the cells. I have read that it dissolves additives and animal hormones added to meats which collect at the joints in humans and can cause arthritic pains. Taking oxygen dramatically stimulates the immune system, increases vitality and maintains good health.

It is safe, can do no harm, and with the level of contaminants in our everyday environment, every man, woman and child in the world could benefit from taking it. Every night before bed and each morning I squirt my mouth with 3 percent hydrogen peroxide, allow it to foam and spit it out.

You may find that oxygen acts as a cure-all, and if it does, that is fine. This does not mean that you should use oxygen as a cure-all and stop seeing your doctor if you are seeing a doctor for some reason. It is a therapy that is complimentary to every other treatment. I just want to emphasize that this natural therapy can compliment your regular health program, and does not necessarily have to be a substitute for it.

Herbs may be the cure for you. We all know the curative and medicinal properties of herbs. However, some herbs can be toxic, especially if taken on a prolonged basis. Herbs are so thoroughly healing and complicated that they are prescribed by doctors in some countries. Vegetable enzymes benefitted everyone and improved every health condition.

One of the safest ways to take herbs is in the form of herbal teas. You can consult with me or a naturopathic physician for help. I have found many people harming themselves by taking toxic herbs far longer than they should.

American Association Of Naturopathic Physicians
818 18th St NW suite 250
Washington DC 20006
(202) 237-8150

American Association of Naturopathic Physicians
Their direct line from the Washington, DC area is: 202-244-1978

Smile Herb Shop (They have an herbalist on staff)
4908 Berwyn Road
College Park, Maryland 20915 phone 301-474-8791

National Center For Homeopathy
801 N. Fairfax St. #306
Alexandria, Virginia 22314 phone 703-548-7790

The National Center For Homeopathy sells a directory for 5 dollars that contains homeopathic as well as naturopathic physicians.

American Institute For Homeopathy
1585 Glencoe
Denver, Colorado 90220

Chapter 22

101 WAYS TO HEAL
THE BODY NATURALLY

When I eat I imagine that my food is super food and that it is making my body super disease-resistant. This kind of mental imaging has been proved to be highly effective in healing the body. Control groups, people who actively imagined their tennis and basketball games improving showed a 25-35 percent improvement. Cancer patients who were told to imagine killer cells going after their cancer had significantly larger numbers of T-cells in their bodies than those that did not go the imaging. There was the case of a nine year old boy who was told that he had a malignant brain tumor and that he only had a few months to live.

When his doctors found, a few months later, that his tumor had completely shrunk they were astonished. He told them that each night when he was put to bed, he sent healing rays to the tumor. The healing rays healed him. The doctors have not figured out <u>how</u> this therapy worked, yet, it does work.

I do something similar to this with my acupressure work. When someone ill comes in and I touch them with my hands, I can always feel the illness in their bodies. For example, I can discern where a headache is by touch. My fingers start to pulse and vibrate as I touch the illness and the swelling and toxins start to dissolve and break up. The electromagnetic energy from my body applied as Acupressure and Shiatsu helps heal the person.

Sometimes when people are being healed they go into a twilight-zone state where they flail their arms and writhe as the toxins leave their bodies. They look much like someone having an epileptic seizure.

They seem to be in a state of hypnosis and are never aware of this altered state. When they awaken, they are totally drunk. Sometimes, they have completely forgotten where they are or who they are for a few seconds upon initially waking.

Now I rarely get sick, but whenever I feel myself getting ill, I touch myself in the place where there is pain and it usually goes away. I figure out what is bothering me emotionally. I get myself into the sunshine and imagine that I am at the bottom of a vat of golden healing rays that are swirling around me and healing me deep inside every pore of my body. I can even feel the soft, gentle air from these rays, for I make them real in my mind. And I get well.

Norman Cousins was told that he had cancer and would die. He checked himself out of the hospital, went out and rented a bunch of comedy videos. He kept watching comedies and his cancer went away. At any rate, he is still alive, and that was years ago. I suspect a few things were at work here. The endorphins from all the laughing and his belief that he could be cured played an important role.

Aromatherapy

Years ago I read an article about the use of aromas to relieve headaches, PMS, tension, emotional distress, stress, lower blood pressure and produce endorphins and a sense of ecstasy. This is now called Aromatherapy. I had been experiencing ecstasy from aromas all my life, and I was struck that I undulated to this innately without knowing or caring why.

I discovered that as we breathe in airborne odor molecules activate receptors in our noses which are turned into nerve impulses which go rapidly to the olfactory bulbs of our brains! It all happens in a second! The olfactory bulbs are the seat of sexual arousal, memory and emotions.

Still the fact that aromas were powerful enough to do all those things amazed me. I tried it out and it's true! Every time I walk into Brookside Gardens at the Wheaton Regional Park in Rockville and smell 2,000 Freesias and Narcissus blooming, I experience heaven on earth (in February and March). I am awash in vivid memories of glorious Easter pageants on hot afternoons with the church full of Freezia, Narcissus and Easter lilies. The smell of Baby's Breath transforms me into a little girl in my grandmother's front yard. They give me a high that is rapturous and like no other experience in life.

It put me in ecstasy to have several pots of blooming Freesias or Narcissus in my bedroom. Yet all that time, I never really understood why. I did know it was worth the 20 dollars to have the blissful lifting delicate scent of the flowers as guests for three weeks. Fresh cut honeysuckles also send my endorphins flying all over the place. Just a few of the plants make my room a paradise of delightful scent. I can work for ten hours with a smile on my face.

Sleeping with the smell makes my sleep restful and my dreams a whole lot nicer. An inexpensive way to experience aromatherapy is to buy

Aromatherapy

the natural extracts from health food stores and place a few drops on the light bulb before turning the light on. Sprinkle a few drops on a damp cloth and put it in the room vent. Sprinkle a few drops on a pan of water that you brought to a boil. The most benefit can be derived from inhaling the fumes directly. The room will become filled with your favorite scent, cushioning and lightening your fun or work.

Many of the aromatic oils are healing. Check with your local herb shop. Some common ones are Cinnamon, Eucalyptus, Lavender and Thyme oils for sinus problems and bronchitis. Juniper oil is used for arthritis. Rosemary oil helps muscle aches. Since the oils are much more concentrated and easily absorbed through the skin, do not use in large amounts.

Put your favorite scent in your bath, among your sheets and linens, closets and underwear. Your favorite smell and your favorite music and color cause your body to make the pleasure hormones that heal and create a space for peace and harmony to occur!

Color Therapy

The Luscher Color Test is a book I stumbled upon in the library that changed my life. In it you will find eight colors. Choose the ones you like in order of preference. Then read Luscher's psychoanalysis of you according to the colors you chose and you will be amazed at how accurate he is.

Discovering Luscher pointed out to me the importance of color in my life. I had always known but never understood the importance of color. I am mesmerized by beautiful flowers, especially the iridescence of Impatiens in the sun. It feels as if I absorb the colors or that they nourish me and affect my consciousness in some way. I discovered that they nourish my body, mind and soul and have an effect on health, how we think and our moods. If you like one or two colors in particular and don't understand why, it probably has a lot to do with how they make you feel.

Photoreceptors in our eyes enable us to see colors. Color in turn activates the pineal and pituitary glands. These glands regulate hormones and we are discovering more everyday how they regulate other bodily systems. Color has been discovered to be a powerful form of energy that can affect many essential life processes and which can heal, soothe, stimulate and produce a variety of effects.

Since color has a tremendous effect on mood, keep that in mind when you choose the colors for your surroundings.

Color therapy is a wonderful way to heal yourself. I found a beautiful old stained glass window that I put up in my window so that the sun can shine through the colors on me. I can feel the yellow and green rays as they stimulate and heal me. If I become too stimulated, I cover the red panels, for they raise blood pressure. Red also warms, excites and energizes. Stay away from it if you have high blood pressure. Notice this the next time you wear red and go under a light or in the sun.

Wear green in the sun to heal yourself. Green has a soothing and healing effect on the body and mind. It lifts depression and anxiety.

Yellow calms and at the same time stimulates pleasantly. It is the most beneficial color for helping the memory. Since it stimulates, it raises blood pressure, lifts spirits and energizes. It is also good for depression and anxiety.

Color Therapy

Black on cold days absorbs the sun, keeping you warmer in cold weather. White reflects it, keeping you cooler on hot days. Blue soothes, and is therefore used to help people relax. Studies show that it reduces blood pressure, respiration and heart rate. It also has a cooling effect.

Orange helps eliminate fatigue and boosts the appetite. It also lifts depression and spirits. Pink is the soothing color. Even the most violent and aggressive individuals have responded positively to pink surroundings. When I want to feel calm and serene, I wear my pink sweater.

The Pineal Gland

The pineal gland is one of the most important hormone-producing glands of the endocrine system. It regulates aging, cyclic activities related to sunlight and seasons, electromagnetic fields, metabolism, behavior and essential assimilative functions of the body. In addition, it regulates blood pressure, body temperature, sleep habits and growth. One of the most important functions of the pineal gland is controlling lymphocyte production. It also controls body temperature, growth, the reproductive system and essential cellular processes.

In order to stimulate the endocrine glands allow sunlight to fall on your eyes for one or two minutes a day. This stimulates the production of important hormones, some of which are very important in aging and agelessness.

Stress sends a distress message to your brain, pituitary and adrenal glands. If you have a vitamin deficiency, your adrenals cannot make the hormones necessary for proper functioning of your body. Often when this happens, allergies emerge.

Also, when your body is stressed, whether the cause is allergic, climatic, infectious, emotional or physical, the adrenals are affected. When the adrenals perform, they secrete cortisol and epinephrine, the fight-or-flight chemicals. If you are deficient in vitamins, minerals and amino acids, you become deficient in adrenal hormones. Feedback between the adrenals and the hypothalamus is critical for the formation of sex hormones. If there is a deficiency or interference from some other source, all of these functions are in jeopardy.

We talked about the massive oil spills that have occurred in our civilized times. How many people know just how harmful it is to ingest petroleum products? This pollutant confuses the body and interferes with the proper functioning of our hormones in addition to contributing greatly to cancer and other degenerative diseases. Within the last five years, I have never seen shrimp or crabs in the shell that did not have oil on their shells!

A major factor that contributes to degenerative diseases today is exposure to petroleum byproducts which are stored by our bodies in fatty tissues. They stay here until the body detoxifies them, and then they are excreted by the liver. An overload of petroleum byproducts would cause nausea, exhaustion, sleeplessness, little aches and pains and depression. Large amounts can cause death.

Of all the magnets that are out there, there is only one that really works. I sell it to my patients. It can prolong your life indefinately. Every illness responds to it.

Natural & Homeopathic Remedies

If you are under a doctor's care, the natural remedies listed below are not known to interact harmfully with over-the-counter medications and prescription medications. However, it is recommended that you do not mix them, but take natural meds two hours after doctor's meds. Homeopathic remedies are in italics. For a more thorough list of ailments and remedies, check the Homeopathic Materia Medica of your favorite homeopathic pharmacy. Using one or a combination of several of the remedies listed should bring relief. Taking oxygen refers to the many successes obtained by people who have cured themselves of chronic diseases using it in the simple manner described in Chapter 20.

Acne	Skin mites cause all acne, delete them. Oxygen, no dairy, no sugar, carrot juice, multiple vitamins and minerals, amino acids from foods (beans, eggs, seeds, nuts) or supplements, an egg a day for the sulphur amino acids, B_6, zinc, Use my Rose Cream, Retin-A or alpha hydroxy acids, eat 70% of diet as fruits and vegetables. Homeopathic acne medicine, B_6, 6 glasses of distilled water a day. Exercise, meditate, acupressure, drink aloe vera juice. *Kali Bichromicum, Sulphur*. Yellow dock and Sarsaparilla tea, Colloidal silver
Addiction	Acupuncture. Prostaglandins (PGE1) (messengers of pain which are blocked by aspirin). For alcohol addiction, AAA. The herb kudzu root reduces desire for alcohol 50 percent in many cases. People report eliminating skin mites reduces addictions
Aggression	No corn, eggs. Take tryptophan, serotonin, niacin, magnesium. Often results from vitamin and mineral deficiency and mites. Multiple vitamins and minerals, mega B-complex
AIDS	Colloidal silver, International Bio-Oxidative Medicine Foundation, PO Box 13205, Oklahoma City, OK 73113, phone 405-478-4266 for a doctor who can give you oxygen therapy. *Mercurius*. See page 169.

Natural & Homeopathic Remedies

AIDS-Related

Allergies — No dairy, no sugar. Oxygen, Colloidal silver, multi. vit. & mineral, which includes B_6, pantothenic acid, 1 to 5 proteolytic, or protein-digesting enzyme tablets & 1 to 2 hydrochloric acid tablets calcium, zinc. Take vitamin C, papaya or papain. Flower remedies: Clematis, Mimulus, Impatiens, Rescue Remedy. *Belladonna, Euphrasia, Apis, Arsenicum, Nux Vomica, Sabadilla.* Some Allergens: Dairy, soy, corn, yeast, wheat, egg products, citrus, chocolate, cinnamon, food coloring, preservatives, fish, shrimp. A reliable test: if heart beats 15 to 20 beats faster thirty minutes after eating a food, allergy to it is certain. (Dr. Cocoa's test)

Aluminum Toxicity — Linked to Alzheimers. Avoid aluminum cookware, it leaches into tomato dishes. Avoid antacid pills. *Carbo veg*, Colloidal silver, chelated minerals

Alzheimer's — Multiple vitamins and minerals,, vitamin C, calcium, magnesium, zinc, B-complex, healthy diet. No aluminum cookware. No antacids with aluminum, kill mites

Anemia — Kill mites, iron from foods like grapes, berries, suma raisins, organic liver, whole grains, green veggies, beans, seeds. Take vitamin C, folic acid, B-complex

Anorexia — B-complex, zinc, magnesium, potassium, *Natrum mur*

Anti-convul-sants — (First speak to a homeopath about symptoms) *Belladonna, Chamomila, Calcarea carbonica, Helleborous, Opium, Stramonium, Nux vomica & Zinc*

Anti-depres-sant — Vigorous aerobic exercise for 30 minutes everyday, multi vitamin and mineral, B-complex. Eat balanced meals. Rose cream

Natural & Homeopathic Remedies

Anti-septics Thyme, Bearberry, Yarrow (not if pregnant), Oxygen, Peppermint, Acidophillus, Chlorophyll, garlic, Rose cream, Colloidal silver

Antisocial Behavior Usually result of gross vitamin/mineral deficiency and mites. Large doses of B-complex for 6 weeks (4-500 mg timed-release per day) then 1-300 mg/day. Multiple vitamins and minerals, amino acids. B_{12}, oxygen. Proper diet. Carrot juice

Anxiety Mega B-complex. No sugar, eggs, artificial flavors. Multiple vitamins and minerals, B_{12} & folic acid shots, calcium & magnesium amino acid chelate, B-complex. Rescue Remedy. *Chamomile, Ignatia*

Arterio-sclerosis Hi zinc to calcium. Massage. Low-fat diet, omega-6 fatty acids pills for 4 weeks, linoleic acid. No alcohol, sugar, milk, lard or butter. Vitamin E, 300 mg/day. Multiple vitamins and minerals, B-complex. Lecithin, alfalfa, pectin, raw garlic. Exercise 3-4 times week

Arthritis Kill mites which cause it, Rose cream, Colloidal silver, vitamin and mineral, vitamin C, 50-1000 mg/day until relieved, B-complex. 400 mg vitamin E/day. Aspirin & copper gluconate together. Carrot juice. Lots of oranges, pineapples and grapefruit. No sugar, white flour. Massage, proteolytic enzymes. *Bryonia, Rhus Tox, Ruta, Pulsatilla* Other natural treatments: alfalfa, wheat grass, watercress, potatoes, yams, celery, parsley, garlic, comfrey, endive, bananas, pineapples, sour cherries & sour apples

Asthma Calcium, oxygen, B_6, vitamin C, 50-3,000 mg over an extended period during an attack, B_{12}, multiple vitamins and minerals, exercise if possible. No dairy, sugar. Take Adrenal gland tablets, pantothenic acid 500-1,000 ml, niacin. *Aconite, Album, Arsenicum, Cuprum Metalicum, Phosphorus Belladonna, Apis, Allium cepa, Euphrasia*, homeopathic

Arthritis Oxygen, magnesium, manganese & zinc, exercise, if poss. 5 or 6 sections from a bulb of raw garlic (on food), kill mites, carrot juice

Asthma Kill parasies, which cause it. Calcium, oxygen, B_6, vitamin C, 50-3,000 mg over an extended period during an attack, B_{12}, multiple vitamin and mineral, Colloidal silver, Rose cream

Natural & Homeopathic Remedies

Backache
Calcium, Yoga, massage. *Arnica, Bryonia, Rhus Tox*

Bacterial Infections
Aconite, or *Belladonna* with Echinacea, Astragalus or Dandelion. Oxygen. Find source of anxiety, Rose cream frustration. Colloidal silver. Lymphatic cleansing

Bad Breath
Chlorophyll, wheat grass, parsley, alfalfa, pancreatic granules, acidophilus, oxygen

Birth Defect Prevention
Multiple vitamins and minerals, mega B-complex, amino acids, load up on fruits and veggies, garlic, oxygen, Coenzyme Q_{10}, organic germanium, organic tofu for protein. No alcohol, caffeine, extended vigorous exercise or hot baths. Keep meticulously clean. Have germ-free sex at all times. Reduce stress. Gently massage your child while pregnant

Bladder Problems
Colloidal silver, oxygen, celery juice, cranberry juice, carrot juice, watermelon. See a homeopathic doctor or pharmacist

Boils
Arsenicum, Belladonna, Hepar Sulphuricum, Silica, Rhus tox, Mercurius, Lachesis. Oxygen, Colloidal silver compress, 3% Hydrogen peroxide compress

Breast Cancer Prevention
Eliminate skin mites which cause it. Oxygen, Colloidal silver, vitamin C, beta carotene, cantaloupe, citrus fruits, kiwi fruit, mango, papaya, carrot juice, broccoli, cabbage, brussels sprouts, Echinacea, no caffeine. Exercise. Homeopathic medicines to boost immune system. Melatonin, vegetable enzymes, acupressure, use Rose cream on self and mate

Blisters
Colloidal silver compress, 3% hydrogen peroxide compress, *Calendula,* applied as a lotion.

Breast Cysts
Eliminate mites, Rose cream, potatoes, oxygen, sesame seeds, cooked apples, cooked mushrooms. Kelp, 3-400 mg of timed-release B-complex daily, vitamin E, zinc, multiple vitamins and minerals. Vegetable enzymes. No caffeine, chocolate, soft drinks, tea. Exercise. Homeopathic Echinacea, Colloidal silver

Natural & Homeopathic Remedies

Bronchitis — No milk, dairy, sugar, corn, soy, formaldehyde (in fabrics, shampoos), yeast, chlorine, wheat, eggs, tetracycline. Take Vitamin C, vitamin A, Thymus gland extract. Oxygen. *Aconite, Kali Bichromate, Pulsatilla*

Bruising — Vitamin C, bioflavonoids, vitamin K, low doses of vitamin E, Acupressure, if used immediately, can prevent bruising

Burning Feet — B-complex, 100 mg timed-release twice a day. Massage

Burns — Crushed ice or something cold immediately for first two or three hours, 20 minutes on/off. For minor burns aloe vera, internally and externally, oxygen, vitamin E oil or raw onion slices or juice on burn. Zinc supplements along with a high protein diet will heal it faster

Bursitis — Massage. No sugar, white flour. Plenty of fresh fruits and vegetables. Oxygen, B-complex twice a day. Vitamin C, calcium/magnesium, proteolytic enzymes

Cancer — Kill parasites, Oxygen, Hospital Santa Monica 619-428-1146 zinc, fresh whole organic foods, organic liver, large amounts of freshly squeezed carrot and orange juices, kelp, bovine colostrum, exercise, if poss. Get rid of all negative thoughts, anger and frustration. High fruit & veg diet, massive amounts of garlic (1 whole clove/day after making sure you are not sensitive to it). Stewed tomatoes. Multiple vitamins and minerals, vitamin C, amino acids. Colloidal silver, vegetable enzymes, Avoid beef, pork, saturated fats, caffeine, chocolate, pollutants, pets, smoking. Take pancreatic enzymes. Rose cream

Burns — Ice immediately, cortisone cream, prescr. strength best, *Mustard Gas, Cantharis, Rhus Tox, Kali Bichromicum,* 30c of either or all

Cancer Prevention — Oxygen, Colloidal silver, carrot juice, beta carotene, vitamin C, multiple vitamins and minerals, amino acids, exercise, peace, organic germanium, Coenzyme Q_{10}, kiwi fruit, low stress, love, kill parasites, enzymes *Belladonna, Bryonia, Phosphorus*

Natural & Homeopathic Remedies

Candida	Oxygen, My Rose cream, acidophilus, Colloidal silver, The Candida Diet or the one in this book. Eliminate fruits for the first 3 months. Massive amounts of raw garlic if you can tolerate it, exercise essential, germanium, Coenzyme Q_{10}
Carpal Tunnel Syndrome	B_6, 1-300 mg/day for 3-4 wks. Vitamins C, and E. Massage
Cataract Prevention	Vitamin E, 400 units/day. Vitamin C, timed-release B-complex. Cystine and methionine
Chicken Pox	*Rhus tox, Pulsatilla, Antimonium tart, Antimonium crudum, Arsenicum, Belladonna & Mercurius,* Colloidal silver
Chicken Pox (Lingering Symptoms of)	Varicellinum, Colloidal silver

Childbirth	To reduce childbirth time and decrease abnormal labor *Caulophyllum, Actea raemosa, Arnica, Pulsatilla, Gelsemium,* 5c
Deliriousness, flushing	*Belladonna, Cimicifuga*
To help turn a breech	*Pulsatilla*
Strengthen uterus for labor	*Caulophyllum (12-30/day during last 2-3 wks of pregnancy*
After delivery for mother and baby	*Arnica*
Caesarean	*Staphysagria*
Long or hard labor	*Sulphur*
Torn perineum	Bellis perrenis 200c, Calendula tincture salve to tear, *Colloidal silver* compress
Asphyxiated	*Antimonium tart* (Even if baby appears dead, it could revive him) *Carbo Veg*

Natural & Homeopathic Remedies

If baby appears blue, cold or unconscious	Carbo veg, camphor, opium
If baby has a facial twitch while gasping for air	Laurocerasus
Baby had traumatic delivery	Arnica, Opium
Neonatal Jaundice	Ck with homeopathic dr. with symptoms for correct remedy. *Aconite, nux vomica, Chelidonium, Lycopodium, Chionanthus, Bovista, or Natrum sulph*
Cholesterol, High	Low-fat diet, omega-6 fatty acids pills for 4 weeks, linoleic acid. No alcohol, sugar, milk, lard or butter. Vitamin E, 300 mg/day. multiple vitamins and minerals, B-complex. Liquid lecithin, alfalfa, pectin, raw garlic. Exercise 3-4 times/week, minimum. Carrot juice. Massage. *Chelidonium, Arnica,* olive oil, enzymes
Chronic Viral Infections	Oxygen. My Rose Cream, Germanium, garlic, *Carbo vegetabalis, Hypericum, Aconite,* Massage. Colloidal silver, Echinacea, exercise, meditation, enzymes
Cirrhosis	Kill liver flukes, Coenzyme Q_{10}, amino acids, liquid lecithin, (very important) milk thistle, dandelion tea, B_{12}, Colloidal silver, mega vitamins and minerals
Cold Hands & Feet	B-complex, 1,000 mg B_3, and calcium/magnesium. Aerobic exercise
Colds	*Colloidal silver, Aconite, Allium cepa, Apis, Euphrasia, Gelsemium, Natrum mur.* Sudaphed at the first symptom will often prevent colds
Colic	*Bryonia, Chamomilla, Pulsatilla, Arsenicum, nux vomica, Magnesia phosphorica, Colocynthis, Lycopodium & Sulphur,* breast milk

Natural & Homeopathic Remedies

Mastitis (inflam-
mation of the *Belladonna, bryonia, phytolacca & lac caninum*
breast

Colitis   Usually a sure cause: dairy products. No dairy, white
              flour, processed sugar. 1-2,000 mg vitamin C/day. Hi
              B-complex, calcium, magnesium, zinc

Common
Cold   Oxygen, *Allium cepa, Euphrasia, Natrum mur, Aconite,*

Concen-   Hi B-complex, lecithin, L-Glutamine, exercise, kill
tration   mites, magnesium, massage, amino acids, Ginko Biloba

Confusion Oxygen, calcium, magnesium, fiber & garlic. Hi B-
              complex, mega vitamins and minerals, vitamin C, 400 mg
              Vitamin E/day. Kill mites. A good diet with nuts,
              seeds, raw vegetables, fruits. Massage. Ginko Biloba

Congestive
Heart   Hi quality organic foods cleaned correctly, oxygen,
Failure   multiple vitamins and minerals B-complex, exercise, if
              possible. Kill parasites. Enzymes, Colloidal silver

Consti-   12 oz. of water upon arising, No milk, dairy. vitamins
pation   and minerals, 50% of diet raw vegs, fruits, sprouted
              grains, nuts, flax seeds, 6 glasses water/ day.
              Purizone (pg. 151) *Bryonia, Aluminia, Nux Vomica, Silica*

Convul-   No sugar, no junk. Taurine, Glutamic acid. Calcium &
sions   magnesium. B-complex, folic acid. Zinc, 30 mg/day.
              Ginko Biloba. No Hyssop, kill mites

Coronary
Heart   Kill mites, Low-fat diet, omega-6 fatty acids pills
Disease   for 4 weeks, linoleic acid. No alcohol, sugar, milk, lard
              or butter. Vitamin E, 300 mg/day. Multiple vitamins
              and minerals, B-complex. Lecithin, alfalfa, pectin, raw
              garlic, pineapple, bananas, oranges, tomatoes,
              potatoes. Exercise 3-4 times week. Colloidal silver

Coughs   Get homeopathic combination, massage. *Bryonia,
              Causticum, Hepar Sulphuris, Kali Bicromium or Spongia*

Cramping   Exercise, *Mag phos, Colocynthis*

Natural & Homeopathic Remedies

Cystic Fibrosis
Selenium, 20-300 mcg, vitamin E, 100-800 units, zinc, 25-50 mg, vitamin C, multiple vitamins and minerals, B-complex

Cystitis
Cystitis, Aconite, Cantharis, Apis, Sarsaparilla

Degenerative Diseases
Oxygen, Colloidal silver, Rose cream, enzymes, Vitamin C, vitamin E, selenium, multiple vitamins and minerals,, B-complex, 300 mg/day, pantothenic acid, 1,000 mg/day, magnesium oxide, 300 mg 3 times/day

Delinquent Behavior
Kill mites. Proper diet, multi. vit & min, amino acids, celery, apple juice, exercise, massage, meditation

Dental Pain
Arnica 7c, *Hypericum* 15c

Depression
Magnesium, B_3, B_6, folic acid, B_{12}, super minerals, multiple vitamins and minerals,s. Depression cannot exist if you exercise. Eat properly. *Arsenicum, Ignatia, Sepia, Pulsatilla, Aurum*

Diabetes
Most important: 40 mcg. chromium/day along with Colloidal silver may eliminate your diabetes. Zinc, Manganese, 3-5% of diet can be fat. Complex carbohydrates, whole grains, potatoes, beans, peas, multiple vitamins and minerals, hi B-complex, super minerals, exercise. No sugar, chips. *Phosphorus. Exercise important. Inositol.* Constantly check new advances through American Association of Diabetic Educators

Diarrhea
Can be a sign that the body is ridding itself of toxins. *Aconite, Arsenicum Album, Veratrum Album*

Ear Infection
Belladonna, Chamomilla, Pulsatilla, Ferrum phos, Hepar sulph

Eczema
Caused by mites, Rose cream, calcium, B_6, vitamin C, B_{12}, multi vit. & mineral, an egg a day for the sulphur amino acids, oxygen, Retin-A or alpha hydroxy acids. *Arsenicum, Graphite, Sulphur, Rhus Venc*

Natural & Homeopathic Remedies

Fever (Infants)	Belladonna, Aconite, Colloidal silver
Fibrositis (Rheumatological)	Treat mites, *Rhus tox* 6c, oxygen
Flu/ Influenza	Colloidal silver, most renowned for flu control: *Anas barbariae hepatica cordis* 200c (commonly marketed as Oscillococcinum), *Gelsemium, Bryonia, Rhus tox, and Eupatorium perfoliatum, Hepar sulph, Apis, Graphities,*
Gallstones	*Celidonium, Berberis, Podophyllum*
Gas, Bloating, Indigestion	Pancreatic digestive enzymes, papaya, B_{12}, folic acid, kill parasites
Gout	*Belladonna, Colchicine*
Grief	*Ignatia*
Hair Loss/ Growth	Kill parasites, Silicone-rich plants: alfalfa, comfrey, young horsetail, common nettle, onions, kelp, oats, buckwheat, barley. Zinc, biotin, multiple vitamins and minerals, vitamin C, mega minerals, B_6, an egg a day for the sulphur amino acids.
Hamstring Injuries	*Ammonium muriaticum*, massage
Hay Fever	Kill parasites, Calcium, B_6, vitamin C, B_{12}, Mineral, Adrenal gland tablets. *Arsenicum Album*, Euphrasia,
Headache	Water, Acupressure, *Arnica, Sanguinaria, Spigelia, Iris, Natrum Muriaticum, Pulsatilla, Gelsemium, Sepia, Belladonna, Chamomilla,* Six glasses of water/day, a banana/day, calcium/magnesium, 1,000 mg vitamin C/day
Heart Attack Prevention	Low doses of chromium, eat bananas, mangoes, apricots. No fat, no sugar. Important: Take vitamins E, C & magnesium, potassium, beta carotene, liquid lecithin. Regular exercise. Kill parasites

Natural & Homeopathic Remedies

Herpes At first onset of a coldsore on lips (A coldsore on the rim of the lip is herpes simplex) soak cotton ball with hydrogen peroxide. Tape to coldsore for several hours. Will suck the virus out of your system and it should not recur. Do not kiss anyone while your zoyster is Hypericum, Kalmia, Magnesia phosphorica, Causticum, Mercurius, Arsenicum

High
Blood
Pressure   Kill parasites, orange juice, tomatoes, potatoes, squash, strawberries, raspberries, blueberries, carrot juice, oxygen, multiple vitamins and minerals

Hives   Kill parasites, *Urtica urens, Apis*

Hyper-
activity*Argenticum nitricum, Arsenicum, Phosphorus, Hepar sulphur, Tuberculinum, Sulphur, staphysagria, Nux vomica & Zinc*

Increase Sexual
Vitality   Oxygen, Kindness, Acupressure, Amino Acids, especially L-Arginine, B-complex, 400 mg vitamin E/day, vitamin C, multiple vitamins and minerals, Ginseng(not if heart weak). Imp. 30-50 mg. manganese. Gotu Kola, Ginseng, Anise. The Better Sex Video Series 1-800-888-1900

Indigestion   Caused by parasites, *Arsenicum Album, Carbo Vegetabilis, Ipecacuanha*

Infections   *Oxygen, Colloidal silver, Aconite, Ferrum phos, Belladonna, Camphora,* Echinacea, Astragulus, Dandelion. Find source of anxiety, frustration. (Remember, see a physician if symptoms persist for more than 2 days)

Inflam-
mation Oxygen. Vitamin C, garlic, Dandelion, digestive enzymes, *Aconite, Apis,* aloe vera, massage

Injuries   *Arnica, Apis.* Massage. Rose cream. With a hematoma use *Bellis perennis,*

Natural & Homeopathic Remedies

Injuries (With
Shooting Pains) *Hypericum*, Rose Cream, apply Colloidal silver

Insomnia   Caused by parasites. Allow your mind 1 hour to disengage from the day's activities. Once in bed clear your lungs by breathing as described on pg. 214. Regular massages prevent it. A massage before bed guarantees an exquisite night's sleep. Take a walk, warm bath or have sex at bedtime. Magnesium/Calcium Amino Acid, B-complex before bed. No caffeine, Sugar, white flour. *Chamomile, Coffea, Ignatia, Nux Vomica* Celery apple juice, exercise, multiple vitamins and minerals. Amino acids. Massage, meditation, Melatonin before bed.

Hyper-
tension Calcium/Magnesium, Coenzyme Q_{10}, follow diet in this book, exercise, mins. Cayenne, Chamomile , fennel, hawthorn berries, rosemary, garlic, Rose Cream, Acupressure

Hypochondria   *Arsenicum*

Irrita-   Kill parasites, No sugar, eggs, artificial flavors.
bility   multiple vitamins and minerals, mega B-complex, B_{12} & folic acid shots, celery-apple juice, exercise, Amino acids. Massage, meditation. Chamomile, *Nux Vomica*, Rescue Remedy

Karposi's
Sarcoma   Phosphorus, Lachesis, Crotalus horridus. Vinblastin 12, Vincristin 12, Bleomycin. Oxygen, Colloidal silver, enzymes,

Lingering   Acupressure
Respiratory
Problems   Oxygen, *Kali bichromium, Kali iodatum, Kali carbonicum, Kali muriaticum, Kali sulphuricum, Silicea, Mercurius, Pulsatilla, Alumina, Nux vomica, Conium*

Liver
Problems   Kill parasites, Colloidal silver, Milk thistle, dandelion, blueberries, raspberries, coffee enema strawberries. No alcohol or drugs. Oxygen, desiccated liver, garlic, choline, Coenzyme Q_{10},

Natural & Homeopathic Remedies

Lung Cancer (Cures only some cases) *Iscador, Viscum Album* (mistletoe, must be homeopathically prepared). Oxygen. Kill lung flukes, Colloidal silver, Acupressure, Hospital Santa Monica 1-800-359-6547

Lung Problems Carrots, parsnips, parsley, celery, mangoes, apricots, the herb Astragalus. Garlic, Coenzyme Q_{10}, germanium, beta carotene, exercise, massage

Memory Problems Increase B_6 until dreams are remembered, then lower dosage. Multiple vitamins and minerals, amino acids, desiccated liver. mega B-complex, Coenzyme Q_{10}, germanium, garlic, amino acids, Ginko Biloba, L-Glutamine

Morning Sickness Colchicum, Sepia, Nux vomica, Silica, Ipecacuaha, Pulsatilla & Symphoricarpus racemosa. Saltines

Menopause Acupressure, *Bryonia, Lachesis, Sepia, Sulphuric Acid* (homeopathically prepared)

Menstrual Problems Acupressure, *Caulophyllum, Colocynthis, Magnesia, Pulsatilla, Sepia*

Muscle Cramps, Aches Magnesium, B_6, vitamin E., C

Nerve Problems Multiple vitamins and minerals, oxygen, mega B-complex, Calcium/magnesium supplement

Osteoporosis Calcium/Magnesium supplement, boron, apples, grapes, pears, 3 glasses boiled whole milk/day

PMS/ Cramping B_6, calcium, magnesium. Aerobic exercise 3 times a week eliminates cramping completely in most cases, folic acid, acupressure, Chamomile & Ginger tea

Post Partum Blues Saint John's Wort

Rocking, Restlessness Calcium, Magnesium

Natural & Homeopathic Remedies

Post-Herpetic Neuralgia — *Hypericum, Kalmia, Magnesia phosphorica, Causticum, Merereum or Arsenicum*

Prophylactics — *Aconite, Ferrum phos, Belladonna, Camphora*

Prostrate Probs — Marshmallow leaves, gravel root and sea holly. Multiple vitamins and minerals, amino acids, zinc, bee pollen, garlic, B-complex

Pus Filled Pimples — Rose cream treatment, Fill cotton ball with H_2O_2 (Hydrogen peroxide), adhere to pimple with removable tape for several hours.

Runner's Knee — *Arnica, Rhus tox, Rhododendron, Ruta, Apis,* massage

Schizophrenia — Kill mites, esp, in head, Oxygen, Zinc, Magnesium, multiple vitamins and minerals, Mega B-complex, Aminos

Sciatica — *Mag phos, Colocynthis,* acupressure

Shin Splints — *Ruta, Rhus tox. Nux vomica and Carbo veg,* alternating doses, Acupressure, Rose cream, Colloidal silver

Shingles — *SRC, Arsenicum, Mezereum, Ranunculus Bulbosus,* oxygen

Smoking — Oxygen, vitamin C, 1-5,000 mg/day, Exercise, High quality foods, Coenzyme Q_{10} multiple vitamins and minerals, B-complex, zinc

Snoring — B_6, vitamin C, B_{12}, Kill parasites

Sore Throat — Gargle with H_2O_2 (3% hydrogen peroxide), preferably food grade) mixed with warm salty water every 2 hours until relieved. Do not swallow. Take *Belladonna, Aconite, Baryta Muriatica, Arsenicum, Rhus tox, Mercurius, Hepar sulph, Lachesis, Apis, Phytolacca*

Natural & Homeopathic Remedies

Sprained Ankle   *Ledum, Arnica*, Colloidal silver compress

Sprains   *Rhus tox, Anacardium, Bryonia or, Arnica.* Zinc for slow healing sprains.

Staphy-
lococcus   *Pulsatilla, Hepar sulph, Apis, Graphities, Staphysagria*

Stimulate Immune
System Exercise 30 minutes, minimum 3x week, Massage, *Carbo veg, Silica* 6c or 10c, Astragalus, Suma, Licorice root (do not use if you have high blood pressure), Ginseng, Goldenseal, Dandelion, Chaparral, Alfalfa, garlic, acidophilus. Mix kelp and the herb thistle seed into salt. Keep teeth and gums are healthy. Rose cream

Tiredness   Oxygen, No dairy, sugar, wheat, eggs, coffee. multiple vitamins and minerals,, B-complex, digestive enzymes, calcium & magnesium, B_{12}, ginseng, bee pollen, aminos

Teething   Belladonna, Chamomilla, Calcarea phosphorica, Calcarea carbonica and Coffea

Throat
Infections   *Belladonna, Arsenicum, Rhus tox, Mercurius, Hepar sulph, Apis, Phytolacca*

Tight
Muscles   *Mag phos*, Magnesium

Toe
Injuries   *Hypericum*

Tranquilizer   Massage, vigorous aerobic exercise for 30 minutes 3 times per week. Melatonin, Rose cream

Ulcers   *Argentum Nitricum, Anacardium, Arsenicum, Nux* Vomica

Varicose
Veins Kill mites which cause them. *Meliotius*

Viral
Infection *Aconite, Ferrum phos, Belladonna, Camphora* (Remember, see a physician if symptoms persist for more than 3 days) Colloidal silver, oxygen, Acupressure

Natural & Homeopathic Remedies

Weak Immune System	Oxygen, acidophilus, germanium, garlic, Coenzyme Q_{10}, amino acids, Multiple vitamins and minerals, mega B-complex, digestive enzymes, *Silicia, Carbo vegetabalis*, Echinacea, Pau d'arco, Red clover, Rhubarb root
Weakness After Flu	*China, Gelsemium, Sulphur, Phosphoricum acidum, Cadmium or Avena sativa*
Weight Loss	Kill mites, watermelon, spirulina, vegetables. Aminos acids and B_{12}. Exercise. Lower fats to 3 percent of your diet. Carbohydrates will give you the energy you normally get from protein. Make sure you get proper proteins from nuts, grains, beans, tofu, green vegetables.
Weightlifters' Stiffness	Massage, Apis, Arnica, Silica

Without plants we would perish as they make the oxygen we breathe and provide us with food. Essential oils and herbs provide medicine from the earth. However herbs are so powerful self medication is not recommended. Essential oils are antiviral, antibacterial, antifungal, antiseptic, antiinflammatory, antineuralgic, antirheumatic, antispasmodic, antivenomous, antidepressant, sedative, digestive, expectorating, stimulate circulation, increase cellular growth and promote healing, bring oxygen and nutrients to tissues, increase electromagnetic frequency and stimulate the body to heal.

Not all natural plants are good for health. Deadly Nightshade is poisonous. Never use essential oils of Bitter Almond, Boldo leaf, Calamus, Devil's claw, Ginseng, Golden seal, Yellow Camphor, Horseradish, Jaborandi leaf, Mugwort, Mustard, Pennyroyal, Rue, Sassafras, Savin, Southernwood, Tansy, Thuja, Wintergreen, Wormseed and Wormwood. If pregnant do not use Basil, Bay leaf, Camphor, Cedarwood, Citronella, Clary Sage, Clove bud, Fennel, Hyssop, Juniper berry, Labdanum, Marojam, Myrrh, Oregano,

Pennyroyal, Peppermint, Rosemary, Sage, Savory, Tarragon, Thyme, Yarrow. Eucalyptus should never be ingested.

Small amounts of the following essential oils are safe during pregnancy: Cardamom, Coriander, Ginger, Grapefruit, Lavender, Lemon, Lemongrass, Lime, Mandarin, Melissa, Neroli, Palmarosa, Petitgrain, Spearmint, Ylang-ylang. It is recommended that no more than five drops of any essential oil be used per day.

The following are known to cause liver damage: Barberry, Comfrey, Golden Ragwort, Groundsel, Huang gin, Mistletoe, Pennyroyal, Sassafras, Scullcap, Senna, Valerian, Wall Germander. Other toxic herbs: Belladonna, Blue Cohosh, Borage, Calamus, Chaparral, Colt's foot, Ephedra (Ma Huang), Germander, Kombucha, Licorice, Lobelia, Magnolia, Poke root, Stephania, Yohimbe. Peppermint and Chamomile can be toxic with prolonged use.

Caffeine is actually a pesticide made by the coffee bean to keep predators away. When humans consume it, the body speeds up and draws water to dilute the poison and quickly eliminates it. This process uses a lot of energy and causes the body to age prematurely. The caffeine speeds up the organs, and thus, wears them out.

Gammahydroxybutyrate (GHB) the body building supplement has proven to be unsafe. Alcohol is addictive, kills brain cells and will burn up the liver and kidneys. Sugar removes calcium from the body, wears out the kidneys and fools the pancreas and gets it out of whack, contributing to diabetes. All meats contain parasites, even organic meats. Animals killed on an assembly line become flooded with uric acid upon seeing the animal ahead killed, knowing he is next. Notice the smell of uric acid in some meats. Sodas contain Phosphoric acid which dissolves paint, flesh and bones and leaches calcium from the body.

Ginseng enhances mental, athletic, immune system and sexual functioning. It increases vitality and aids in stress management. It should not be taken by those with heart problems and for only ninety days at a time.

WHATEVER YOUR HEALTH PROBLEM – WE CAN HELP!

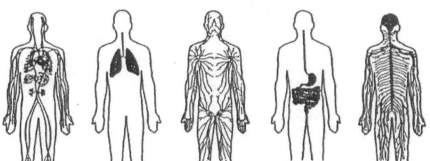

ARTHRITIS ALLERGIES CANCER CANDIDA
HEART DISEASE DIABETES WEIGHT CONTROL

Full Hospital Facilities	or	Resort Spa

Hospital Santa Monica   **Agua Caliente Spa**

Full Hospital Facilities	Resort Spa Atmosphere
9 Physicians	Physicians and Nurses
1 Chiropractor	Chiropractor
1 Dentist	Hot Mineral Water
Physiotherapy	Destressing Program
Colonics	Weight Control Program
Hydrotherapy	Massage
Bio-Magnetic Therapy	Muscle Stimulation
Live Cell Therapy	Live Cell Therapy
Acupuncture	

Alternative Therapies including: Hydrogen Peroxide, Laetrile, Shark Cartilage, Hydrazine, Clodronate, Flutamide, DMSO, Cesium, Thymosin, Interferon, etc. These facilities are under the direction of Kurt W. Donsbach, DC, PhD and offer the most complete wholistic therapy available in the world. Cancer patients have over 20 different proven therapies available to them. Both Hospital Santa Monica and Agua Caliente are sparkling new facilities and are worthy of your most critical evaluation. Please call for a free brochure on both these facilities, including insurance information, charges, and tips on what to bring for your healthful stay at these Baja, Mexico health facilities without the restrictions of the health monopoly present in the U.S. YES THERE IS HOPE!

USA (619)428-1146

Baja Mexico (011)526-613-3333

NATIONAL HEALTH FEDERATION
P.O. BOX 688, MONROVIA, CA 91017
(818) 357-2181

Your Health Freedom is at Risk!
Join NHF NOW!

The National Health Federation is a 39-year-old consumers rights organization, one of the most informed, responsive and effective grassroots organizations in the country. National Health Federation is working to guarantee your right to use the doctor, nutrition and therapy of your choice.

The National Health Federation:
- Encourages natural health preventive therapies over modern drug therapies.
- Fights against the Drug Monopolies/FDA/AMA cronies who want vitamins regulated as drugs.
- Works for the passage of effective health-freedom legislation at the local, state and national levels.
- Advocates to change dangerous legislation, such as forced fluoridation, vaccinations and prescription drugs
- Analyzes legislation and alerts consumers and consumer-action organizations of attempts to take away your freedoms.
- Offers education to consumers on the subjects of natural health.

It is an honor to belong to the National Health Federation whose membership philosophy embraces the traditional, orthodox harmless forms of therapy that were used and taught by Hippocrates, the father of natural therapies. Hippocrates espoused a natural life style and the edict of "first do no harm."

Join Now or Send a Gift Membership to your Friends and Family!

We will send a beautiful gift acknowledgement that will tell your loved ones you really care!

Check, money order or Visa/Mastercard:
Card #_____ Exp. date_____

NHF
- ❑ **$2,000 Perpetual Membership** *(can be willed)*
- ❑ **$1,000 Life Membership**
- ❑ **$100 Sustaining Membership** *(annual)*
- ❑ **$36 Regular Membership**

Name_____

Address_____

City_____ State_____ Zip_____

Please consider making a gift today to support the NHF's work. **Donations accepted on the website: https://squareup.com/store/national-health-federation-3**

Chapter 23

```
┌─────────────────────────┐
│  NOW ANYONE CAN         │
│  LOSE WEIGHT AND        │
│  KEEP IT OFF, FOR       │
│         LIFE            │
└─────────────────────────┘
```

I discovered over the years what causes everyone to be overweight: parasites, usually in the intestines, but skin mites can cause it too. Nothing will help you lose weight like killing the parasites. Another factor that contributes to bulky bodies is combining foods improperly which causes some foods to sit in the stomach and putrefy while others are digested. Then I stumbled upon the laws of natural hygiene which teach how to combine foods so they are properly digested, and I could feel the difference in my body; no more stomach aches or bloated feelings. You will lose weight without starving following the delicious diet described in this chapter. Make sure all raw foods are cleansed as described on pages 79 and 80. Blemishes on fruits usually indicates they have been invaded by an animal or parasite. Eat no raw apples, watermelon, nor raw carrots unless they come clean. When the peroxide stops bubbling, then the vegetables are clean. Never eat unwashed sprouts, as they are loaded with parasites. Nuts and seeds usually have parasites so they must be cleaned.

The diet is very simple. At the beginning of the day eat a fruit meal. This means a pound (or even two if you have a big appetite) of fruit. You need enough to fill you up so that you are not hungry for several hours. For as long as you can, eat fruits and drink extracted fresh fruit and vegetable juices and water until you feel the need for denser food. Do not eat anything else with it.

Sometimes before lunch I will have two of these kinds of fruit meals. I also eat them for midnight snacks.

Do you have a healthy sweetener that you like? Put it on your fruits on those occasions when it is not as sweet as you would like it to be. You can make your fruits come alive with tiny amounts of Vegetable Glycerin or Stevia. There are natural sweeteners made from barley, beets and other natural ingredients.

Small amounts of natural sweeteners sprinkled on fruits can take it from tasteless to exciting. To pick good fruit, smell and color are good indicators of sweetness and succulence. The cut stem of a melon should have the smell of the melon, and likewise with peaches and other fruits. Firm flesh is preferred in most cases.

Eat the fruit in the easiest form for you. Make sure your fruit meals are always delicious and you will always eat them. I cut mine up in a big bowl and eat it over a period of from five minutes to a half an hour. But you may want to liquify yours in the blender or consume the fruit as a milk shake.

Add fresh and frozen fruit, ice or frozen yogurt, low-fat pina colada yogurt and a dab of vanilla extract to make a delicious creamy shake that is easily digestible. Use half-fresh and half-frozen fruit and you get a thick, creamy non-fat shake that will virtually eliminate your craving for ice cream. Except for shakes, the juices you drink should be freshly extracted from the fruits and vegetables. Milk should be boiled slowly for 20 minutes.

Drink within five or ten minutes of extracting or blending as the juices are very fragile. Processing foods this way allows the very essential enzymes from the fruits and vegetables to be used by your body immediately. Enzymes aid in digestion and kill harmful agents. When consumed on a regular basis, freshly squeezed juices and this diet will make your body a superpowered disease-fighting machine!

When you eat an orange, bite into the peeling, which is where the joy of an orange is. The peeling is indigestible, although it will not agree with some. It is best to eat small amounts of orange peeling to minimize indigestion.

For lunch have a soup and salad or fresh vegetables, pasta and baked potato, or have all five.

Make sure you get adequate amounts of amino acids, as they are essential for all bodily functions, Eat small amounts of high quality proteins three times a week. Organic tofu, organic meats (if you eat meat) or supplements such as spirulina contain adequate amounts.

Stop being so careful to make sure you are not hungry all the time. I assure you, your body is not going to allow you to starve.

Do not eat proteins with starches and/or sugars at the same time. Proteins such as nuts, beans, flesh foods and eggs should be eaten together, but separately because of the digestive juices needed to digest them. They can also be eaten with green and low-starch vegetables. Proteins need an acidic medium for digestion. Carbohydrates, which are starches and sugars, need an alkaline medium for digestion.

Dinner can be similar to lunch. Eat enough that you are not hungry. You will lose weight. If you are a meat eater, it is recommended that meats be eaten in small portions two or three times a week. Other sources of protein, grains, beans and vegetables can be used.

The following is reprinted with permission of V.E. Irons. © by V.E. Irons

This is very important. No diet will work if you do not enjoy the food. If your fruits and vegetables are not flavorful or spicy enough, make them that way. It will be impossible for you to reap the benefits of all these healthy, healing whole foods if you do not enjoy eating them, because you will not continue to eat them.

One of the reasons so many diets fail is because the people on them don't love the food. Sweeten fruits by cutting up ripe bananas over them and eat the bananas with the other fruits to sweeten them. The reason this diet works for me is because I am eating foods I love.

The following is reprinted with permission of V.E. Irons. © by V.E. Irons

FOODS IN DETAIL — FOR CHART READING

PROTEINS

(a) **Concentrated**

meat, eggs,
fish, cheese,
poultry and
*milk

(b) **Less Concentrated**

(Vegetable)
nuts, beans,
peas, lentils

VEGETABLES

All vegetables
(except potatoes
and tomatoes as
shown) combine
with all classes —
see center of chart

FRUITS

(a) **Acid**

grapefruit
lemons
oranges
cranberries
tomatoes

(b) **Sub-Acid**

blueberries
raspberries
strawberries
peaches
apples
pears
apricots
cherries
grapes
pineapple
prunes

CARBOHYDRATES

(a) **Starches**

Permissible:
bananas,
potatoes,
cereals, bread,
pies, cakes,
spaghetti
made with
*unbleached whole
grains* with NO
chemicals added

(b) **Sugars**

Permissible:
honey, maple syrup,
raw & dark brown
sugar,
unsulphured molasses,
dried fruits

HYDROCARBONS

Fats

cream
butter
olive oil
peanut oil
soy bean oil
sesame seed oil
sunflower seed oil
lard
animal fats —
sparingly

Avoid

butter substitutes
and all prepared
hydrogenated fats

COMMENTS and EXCEPTIONS

Don'ts . . .

1. DON'T drink MILK and eat MEAT at the same meal.

   *Although milk is a Protein it requires a different digestive medium than concentrated proteins like meat, fish and poultry. The old Mosaic Law made it a SIN to eat milk with meat. Avoid building TOXIC POISONS of UNDIGESTED PROTEINS when meat and milk are used at the same meal since neither may properly digest. USE MILK AS THE ONLY PROTEIN OF THE MEAL, and NOT AS A BEVERAGE with meat.

2. ELIMINATE from the diet ALL PRODUCTS made of refined, white or whole wheat bleached and chemically treated flours synthetically fortified. These "empty calorie" products merely take the place of truly nutritious foods. Use products made from unbleached flour which still contains it's nutritional value. If your intestinal tract can take it use whole grain flours.

3. ELIMINATE ALL REFINED SUGARS and all products pre-sweetened when purchased. They are usually sweetened with white sugar and/or synthetic glucose, which again merely supply "empty calories." Use only honey, maple syrup, raw or dark brown sugar and unsulphured molasses.

4. NEVER COOK ANYTHING you can possibly eat RAW.

5. NEVER eat DESSERTS — except FRUITS.

6. AVOID all MEATS treated with SYNTHETIC HORMONES or CHEMICALS.

7. AVOID all FATS that have been "hydrogenated."

Do . . .

1. Eat a raw VEGETABLE SALAD daily — eat it before starting main course.

2. Eat two or more pieces of FRESH FRUIT DAILY.

3. Eat FRUITS *only* for dessert, preferably raw.

4. Use CONCENTRATED PROTEINS only once daily — less CONCENTRATED PROTEINS anytime.

6. DRINK water heavily between meals — not for two hours after or half-hour before.

7. MELONS are best eaten between meals.

8. Eat a large helping of a cooked LEAFY VEGETABLE daily — for laxative purposes.

9. "EAT NOTHING UNLESS IT WILL SPOIL or ROT but eat it before it does." — Dr. McCollum.

10. EXERCISE — even good balanced blood is ineffective unless aerated (oxygenated) so walk, walk, walk.

11. Condition the mind with POSITIVE THINKING.

12. To help provide elements that might be deficient in your diet we recommend supplementing your diet with the 100% NATURAL FOOD CONCENTRATE made of the DRIED EXTRACTED JUICES of the young green CEREAL GRASSES, OATS, RYE, WHEAT, CORN and BARLEY grown on organically treated soils without chemical fertilizers or poisonous sprays, and commercially known as *greenlife*

NOTE: Various nutritional authorities disagree on best recommended diets. The above suggestions incorporate dietary propositions that have been most successful for a great number of persons in improving their nutrition. Any suggestions are nutritional, only, and are not intended as a substitute for medical treatment of non-nutritional situations.

SPRINGREEN PRODUCTS, INC., Natick, Mass. 01760

LIVING NATURE'S WAY... *Proper Foods... Properly Combined*

As we grow older many of us find we cannot as easily digest or "handle" the vast assortment of conflicting foods that we once did. Why?

Because for too many years we have imposed on our wonderful digestive mechanism in many ways; one of these impositions may have consisted of requiring it to do two opposing operations at the same meal, namely:

Digest *proteins*, which require a strong *acid* medium, and at the same time

Digest *concentrated carbohydrates*, which require an *alkaline* medium.

The CARBOHYDRATES need the *alkaline* saliva of the mouth and the *alkaline* juices of the intestine to complete digestion. The PROTEINS activate the pepsin of the stomach needed to split the protein molecule, and bring forth the hydrochloric acid needed for complete protein digestion. Acids and alkalies when brought together can neutralize each other so that neither type of foods are easily or thoroughly digested. Too frequently this results in *fermentation* of the carbohydrates and *undigested acid end products* from the proteins. All this may tend to add toxins and thus the body's vitality is lowered. When one's digestive system has been weakened it should naturally be given every aid in self recuperation*

Many "so-called" authorities disagree with this proposition, but why theorize or enter into a "scientific" discussion. We believe that you can and should prove its nutritional value yourself.

IF for 30 days you will rigidly avoid WRONG COMBINATIONS OF FOODS YOU WILL UNDOUBTEDLY BE AMAZED at the friendly, contented feeling in your stomach and at your feeling of renewed strength and well being.

Explanation:

For purposes herein we define a product as PROTEIN if it contains fifteen per cent or more PROTEIN, and a product as CARBOHYDRATE if it contains twenty per cent or more starch.

*Man Alive You're Half Dead — D. C. Munro, M.D., pages 72-106, also A New Health Era — Wm. Howard Hay, M. D., pages 76-86.

THIS CHART WITH ITS COMMENTS MAY SUGGEST TO YOU WHAT YOU CAN AND WHAT YOU CANNOT SUCCESSFULLY COMBINE indefinitely.

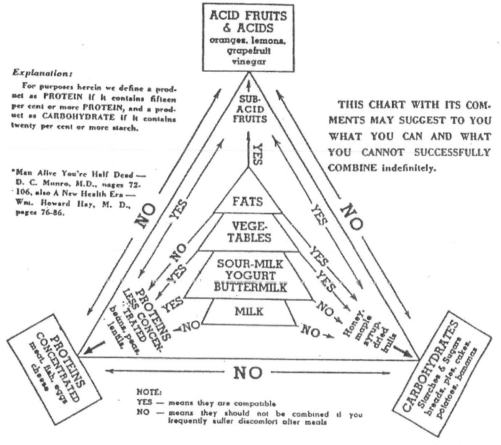

NOTE:
YES — means they are compatible
NO — means they should not be combined if you frequently suffer discomfort after meals

Try This!

To make my body a super-powerful disease-fighting machine I either extract the juices from organically grown fruits like pears, apples, bananas, cherries, blueberries, pineapple, or I liquify them in the blender. I sometimes add a little fresh coconut to make myself a delicious, powerful drink. I vary the fruits, and these drinks are a highlight of my day for they are delicious, soothing and healing.

Please read the testimonials about this product. I think it will help anyone greatly. It is a cell regenerator and much more:

https://supplementpolice.com/niagen/
(Nicotinamide Riboside) Nicotinamide Riboside and Niagen are often celebrated as a "fountain of youth." They have been linked to many health benefits...

This is a brain boosting supplement that helps with memory as well as body regeneration. You can read about it here.
http://www.lifeextension.com/Magazine/2011/2/Generate-Fresh-Mitochondria-with-PQQ/Page-01

This one is with CoQ10 so you can use this one instead of taking two supplements:
https://www.amazon.com/Mitochondria-Maximizer-Peak-Performance-Vegetarian/dp/B075R2XCJV/ref=sr_1_1_sspa?ie=UTF8&qid=1521600505&sr=8-1-spons&keywords=peak+performance+mitochondria+maximizer&psc=1

Fortified Foods Could Fight Off Cancer read the headline in the New York Times.

"For fruit-poor diets, scientists propose anti-cancer foods."[87]

Foods Are Cure For What Ails You

---

[87] © 1991 by The New York Times Company. Reprinted by permission.

"Bananas for ulcers, cranberry juice for bladder infections, pumpkin seeds for prostrate problems, yogurt for vaginal infections, strawberries for headaches and apples for high cholesterol."[88]

The extracted vegetable juice is the only thing that can be drunk with meals (except fruit juice with fruit meals) and while drinking it, hold it in your mouth to allow the digestive juices in your mouth to be absorbed into the juice. You are safe to mix a large variety of fruits when extracting juices, but the rule to follow is that only apples can be mixed with vegetables.

Acidic and alkaline fruits should be eaten separately. See the chart for combining foods. I break the rule sometimes and add fresh beets to my fruit shakes and it does not give me stomachache as it is supposed to. When I cheat I add whipped cream to my fruit. I don't do it very often.

When you eat just the fruit meal, allow the fruit at least thirty minutes, and the vegetables one hour for digestion. I suppose you are worried about this as I was when confronted with the thought of having to measure the time that passes after I have eaten something, but realizing how important it was to my health to do this correctly, I nevertheless committed to doing it.

I suggest a Ketogenic Diet and avoiding toxic lectins in foods. "Ketogenic" means you get your calories from proteins and fats and eat less carbs. The idea is for your brain to run on protein and fats instead of sugar, to cut back on carbs that are quickly digested like sugar, soft drinks, pastries and white bread. Lectins in foods are plant poisons that interfere with our digestion and are largely found in *grains of all kinds, (especially wheat, beans, soy) nuts and dairy and nightshade plants such as eggplant, tomatoes, potatoes and peppers* of all kinds.

It is best to avoid eating proteins with carbs, such as meat on a sandwich. The combination is hard for our bodies to digest. Both require different digestive juices so the carbs with putrefy in your stomach while waiting for the proteins to digest, which can take up to 4 hours. Proteins with low-grade starches like cabbage, cauliflower, broccoli are ok to eat with meats.

---

[88] © 1990 by The Washington Times.

a small amount of protein with veggies. On another occasion, you can have your carbohydrate and vegetable meal.

This point is so important, I must reiterate, *allow four hours for the digestion of proteins, one or two for digestion of carbohydrates and vegetables, at least thirty minutes for fruits and ten minutes for fruit juices and* mineral *water*, which all should be consumed separately.

In some cases you can break the rules. It is important to know what foods can be combined for maximum digestion, and thus, absorption of nutrients. Carbohydrates can be eaten with fruits if you have no ill effect from doing it. Carbohydrates or proteins can be eaten with vegetables, but do not eat carbohydrates and proteins together.

Drink plenty of water or fruit juices, preferably freshly squeezed or extracted, between meals, but drink nothing like beer of soda with meals. If you must consume these drinks, do so between meals so they do not interfere with the absorption of important nutrients. Drinking dilutes the digestive juices, which can cause problems like stomachache, headache, nausea, etc. Watch these problems disappear as you follow this diet.

If I say when drinking structured water or fruit juice allow ten minutes for digestion I mean that you should not eat anything within that ten minute period after you drink it.

The laws of natural hygiene have proven that it is very important how foods are combined. Seventy-five percent of what we eat should be raw foods, preferably fruits and vegetables. Make sure to wash all raw foods in the solution of 3% hydrogen peroxide and baking soda. Only small amounts of protein are needed, and it does not have to be in the form of meat, it can be roasted nuts.

Sufficient amounts of almost everything we need can be found in a variety of organic fruits, leafy green vegetables, fresh squeezed juices, meats and roasted nuts. For your protein meals eat things like soups made with bone broth and lots of concentrated veggies, and little meat or organic whey. You can use coconut flour to thicken. Raw avacado or salad provides needed enzymes and fiber. We advocate following a Ketogenic low-lectin diet. Ketogenic means high-fat, adequate-protein, low-carbohydrate diet that in medicine is used primarily to treat difficult-to-control epilepsy in children. The diet forces the body to burn fats rather than carbohydrates. Normally, the carbohydrates contained in food are converted into glucose, which is then transported around the body and is particularly important in fueling brain-function. However, if there is little carbohydrate in the diet, the liver converts fat into fatty acids and ketone bodies. The ketone bodies pass into the brain and replace glucose as an energy source. An elevated level of ketone bodies in the blood, a state known as ketosis, leads to a reduction in the frequency of epileptic seizures. Almost half of children, and young people, with epilepsy who have tried some form of this diet saw the number of seizures drop by at least half, and the effect lasts even after discontinuing the diet.

It is very important to eat foods that you like. It produces healing endorphins in our bodies. You will eat less and feel more satisfied. A blender and vita mix enable us to enjoy more concentrated foods. However, eating too many concentrated foods like kale, collards, mustards, especially in a smoothie, can give us too many oxylates than our bodies can handle and we end up with a kidney stone. To counter that always take probiotics as they will handle the oxylates and move them safely from the body.

If you eat meat, small amounts of it combined with vegetable such as in Chinese food, form complete proteins. For example, a skillet of stir fried vegetables with small strips of meat can provide enough complete protein for 4-6 people. Even though protein is essential, only small amounts are needed. Too much robs the body of calcium, which can be dangerous. It also puts an overload on the kidneys which have the job of processing protein. Over a long period of time, this can cause health problems.

A healthy alternative is bone broth with onions simmered in it, then add your favorite vegetables and spices like Turmeric, Rosemary, Garlic, Coriander, Cumin to create a healing soup. I keep quarts of organic concentrated soups in my refrigerator at all times as well as fermented veggies such as sauerkraut made with slivered cabbage. Made in large batches, these provide valuable nutrition to form a balanced meal.

I eat massive amounts of raw and cooked garlic everyday (1 or 2 cloves). This is probably one of the best health-promoting herbs that you will find. In fact, it does so many good things for the body, it is considered a super-food. Some people are sensitive to it raw. Make sure you are not one of them.

I add garlic to one of the foods I'm eating. For example, I love it with lemon juice, therefore I eat a lot of guacamole with garlic, cilantro and lemon juice.

Another way to clean your tongue is by spraying 3 percent hydrogen peroxide your toothbrush or a washcloth and washing the candida away.

Pancreatic cancer, is the fifth leading lethal cancer in the U.S. While beta-carotene, selenium, and vitamin E offer some protection, Lycopene protected against pancreatic cancer far better than any other nutrient tested. Only LIFE EXTENSION MIX™ contains lycopene.

Vitamin B-12 has shown anti-cancer benefits, but in order to absorb this vitamin, many people have to take B-12 shots. LIFE EXTENSION MIX™ uses an ion exchange resin which is the _only_ oral method of absorbing vitamin B-12.

In some studies, the fat-soluble form of vitamin C called Ascorbyl Palmitate worked better than water soluble ascorbic acid in preventing cancer and free radical damage to body fat. The LIFE EXTENSION MIX™ formula contains _both_ forms of vitamin C for maximum protection.

Selenium is the most important mineral in a life extension program. Organic and inorganic selenium have different beneficial effects and only LIFE EXTENSION MIX™ contains both.

A debate has been going on for decades as to whether natural or synthetic vitamin E is better. The facts now show the benefits of taking both forms and only LIFE EXTENSION MIX™ has both natural _and_ synthetic vitamin E.

Most free radical damage occurs within the cell in the mitochondria. Sulfur-containing amino acids inhibit this dangerous free radical damage to mitochondria better than any other antioxidants. LIFE EXTENSION MIX™ contains potent doses of these amino acids.

The mutation of a cell is the first step leading to the development of cancer. Certain plant flavonoids have demonstrated an antimutagenic effect that can prevent changes in cells that lead to cancer. Only LIFE EXTENSION MIX™ contains these plant flavonoids.

Daily Dose of LIFE EXTENSION MIX™

		% U.S. RDA
CAROTENOID COMPLEX		
Vitamin A	5000 IU	100
Beta-Carotene	25000 IU	500 of vit A
Lycopene Complex	7500 IU	**
Xanthophyll Complex	7500 IU	**
B COMPLEX		
Vitamin B1 (Thiamine HCl)	250 mg.	16666.67
Vitamin B2 (Riboflavin)	50 mg.	2941.20
Vitamin B3 (niacin 75/niacinamide 100)	175 mg.	875
Vitamin B5 (Calcium Pantothenate)	750 mg.	7500
Vitamin B6 (Pyridoxine HCl)	200 mg.	**
Vitamin B12 (Ion Exchange Resin)	100 mcg.	1666.67
PABA	250 mg.	**
Folate Trigluriamate (folic acid)	800 mcg.	180
Biotin	200 mcg.	66.67
ASCORBATE COMPLEX		
Vitamin C (from calcium, magnesium and niacinamide ascorbates)	2500 mg.	4166
Vitamin C (Ascorbyl Palmitate)	500 mg	354 of vit C
SELENIUM AND TOCOPHEROL COMPLEX		
Sodium Selenate	50 mcg.	**
Seleno-Methionine (Nutr. 21)	50 mcg.	**
Vitamin E (d, l-alpha tocopherol acetate)	300 IU	1000.00
Vitamin E (d-alpha tocopheryl succinate)	300 IU	1000.00
ELECTROLYTE MINERAL COMPLEX		
Calcium Stearate	250 mg.	1.65 Ca.
Calcium Aspartate	150 mg.	3.00 Ca.
Calcium Succinate	150 mg.	3.44 Ca.
Vitamin D3	100 IU	25
Magnesium Chloride	800 mg.	51.06 Mg.
Magnesium Aspartate	100 mg.	2.11 Mg.
Magnesium Succinate	100 mg.	3.63 Mg.
Potassium Aspartate	50 mg.	**
Potassium Chloride	49 mg.	**
AMINO ACID COMPLEX		
L-taurine	500 mg	**
L-cysteine	500 mg.	**
L-glutathione	15 mg.	**
CHOLINERGIC COMPLEX		
Choline Bitartrate	500 mg.	**
Phosphatidyl Choline	150 mg.	**
Inositol	250 mg.	** .
FLAVONOID COMPLEX		
Luteolin Complex	50 mg.	***
Robinetin Complex	100 mg.	***
Myricetin Complex	100 mg.	***
Hesperidin Complex	250 mg.	***
ADDITIONAL NUTRIENTS		
Dilaurylthiodipropionate	25 mg.	***
Thiodipropionic Acid	25 mg.	***
Bromelain	15 mg.	***
Freeze Dried Cabbage Conc.	500 mg.	***
ADDITIONAL MINERALS		
Zinc (picolinate)	15 mg.	100
Zinc (succinate)	15 mg.	100
Chromium (picolinate)	80 mcg.	**
Molybdenum (Sodium Molybdate)	125 mcg.	**
Manganese (gluconate)	5 mg.	**
Iodine (Kelp)	10 mcg.	6.7

** U.S. RDA has not been established.
*** Need in human nutrition has not been established.

Of all the vitamins on the market, this one is the most outstanding.

© 1993 by Life Extension Foundation, PO Box 229120, Hollywood, FL 33022-9120. 1-800-841-5433. Reprinted with permission.

> ### How To Eliminate Your Stomach!

Drink two of the fruit shakes I described and your stomach will shrink, and possibly, disappear. Slowly drink a blender full (about 32 ounces) or half a blender full over a ten minute period. Drink as a meal as it should fill you up for two or three hours. I mix my 32 ounce blender full of fresh and frozen fruits, fortify with liquid lecithin, acidophilus, organic tofu, amino acids, herbs, etc. I drink and eat as much as I want and am never hungry! The fruit you eat can eliminate the craving for sugary items.

When you fill your stomach with healing fruits instead of potato chips and hamburgers, it will be impossible for your stomach to bulge with all that healthy fiber unclogging you. Try the above for two weeks, and you won't believe the difference in how you feel, look and think. If you are overweight, you will lose.

Continue eating this way, and you will never be fat! Another secret to shrinking your stomach is to get enough to drink. Do not go from meal to meal without having at least two glasses of some liquid, preferably water, between. Make sure you get at least six glasses of water or some liquid per day and you will eliminate constipation as well.

Sometimes a cold can be an indication that you are clogging your system up too much with food and not drinking enough. Substitute some of the fruit drinks for meals when you have a cold. Drink more between meals, and you will find your requirement for food diminishing as your stomach shrinks and you lose weight.

Listen to your body. It will tell you gently, then loudly what it needs. Sometimes I can eat fruit and drink juices until late afternoon and not feel hungry.

Get out of the habit of eating on a schedule. Try to never, ever eat unless you're hungry! Unnecessary eating stretches your stomach and throws your entire system off. It is much healthier to eat only when hungry and not according to a schedule.

When you continually force food into a body that is not ready for it, you can throw yourself off balance. As well as I know this rule, I still find myself tempted sometimes to eat on schedule. Example, I look at the clock and think, it's seven hours since I ate. I'm not even slightly hungry. I'm sure I will be getting hungry soon.[89]

Then, an hour later, I'd think, I'd better be getting hungry soon or I might develop one of those hungry headaches. Two hours later, after drinking sixteen ounces of freshly extracted organic carrot, broccoli, cucumber and apple juice, I think, I should be hungry by now, even though I'm not. An hour later, I may still not be hungry enough to eat because I have drank a glass of water.

Then I realized I was obsessing over it! I stopped it. And the paragraph above will, hopefully, prevent you from getting into that. I discovered that if I just went with the flow of the day and simply thought of it as another day that I got to live, and enjoy life, such petty things slipped away. I learned to go with the natural flow of my body and I became so much more in harmony and synchronized. I learned that my body was not going to allow me to starve, and I did not have to worry about it. Magically, the problem disappeared.

If you have any post-nasal drip or any kind of respiratory disease, try eliminating dairy products from your diet and supplement with vitamin C (250-500 mg/day) and you will be amazed at how your respiratory problem will be reduced. It has been discovered that dairy products are mucous-forming and therefore promote mucous formation in our bodies. Allergies and asthma are caused by parasites (see BODY BEASTS in the December 1998 National Geographic Magazine) I have eliminated every case that came to me by simply killing the parasites. Lately there has been a lot in the news about the process used to homogenize milk causing diabetes.

---

[89] Only within the last five years have I realized that I had an unconscious fear of starving, transmitted from my mother. My mother used to go bananas when, as a child I would sometimes go for three days without eating. I realized as an adult that I had gotten a sick pleasure over her distress over me. I slowed the time down so I would not get hungry.

Chapter 24

KEEPING TONED FOR LIFE

Before beginning any exercise program, please notify your doctor and make sure that it is safe to begin. Before I started twenty-five years ago I went in and had a stress test. I was shocked to hear them say that my heart was as strong as a horse's! I had been having chest pains, and thought I was seriously ill. The chest pains went away when I started running.

I discovered later that they were actually from my stressful job situation. I think it is important to clarify why exercise is so important so that it can gain its due respect from the person who wants to use it to enhance and prolong life.

Running, walking, swimming, skiing and trampolining are some aerobic exercises that will stimulate your immune system, slow or prevent aging, strengthen your body and keep your muscles toned. Aerobic exercise is the most efficient way to exercise the heart, one of our most vital organs. It has been proved over and over that people who exercise this vital organ live longer than people who don't.

These kinds of exercises also cause us to breathe fully, which is the only time the immune system operates at maximum capacity. This means that the entire body gets oxygenated, and the high like the one described by runners is possible. During this process of oxygenation, a massive amount of healing, cleansing and purification occurs.

If you lose fifty pounds or even twenty pounds and don't tone, you are going to look like a mass of slack flesh. Worse, you will probably feel like one too. You can keep it simple: jog or do powerwalking for twenty minutes a minimum of three times a week! Stretch and flex your arms as you go. Five to thirty minutes of Yoga a day will make a very noticeable difference in keeping you balanced. Stretching is a good way to tone and firm muscles.

Keeping toned keeps the immune system strong. Meditating, proper nutrition, fresh air and sunlight shining on the skin and eyes, massage, and Yoga are also excellent for strengthening the immune system. Usually anything that pleases us and gives us joy, and almost anything that causes us to breathe deeply and fully oxygenates the body and stimulates the immune system.

The extent of activation and stimulation depends on how long you allow yourself to enjoy what you are enjoying. For example, looking at a beautiful view or smelling your favorite flowers, looking at the face of the one you love, hearing your favorite music, or even Yoga will stimulate the making of soothing, healing, endorphins.

In fact one of the oldest and most common ways of stimulating the immune system and healing the body is Yoga, which is a simple ancient synchronized deep breathing and stretching.

Yoga

Of all the exercises that exist, Yoga is superior to them all for it re-balances mind, body and spirit. Wise men in India discovered long ago that the mind, body and spirit had a tendency to want to go in their own separate directions and a system was needed to re-balance them. Yoga is good for helping to lose weight and keeping it off, firming and toning muscles and eliminating stress and pain. Yoga is also known to bring out the natural beauty in a person. Certainly it adds to a person's grace and poise. It creates calm and a positive outlook.

Yogis believe that life is in the breath and that he who half breathes half lives. We can go without food or water for many days, but we cannot last one moment without air. Since the primary element sustaining life is oxygen, Yoga teaches that a subtle element in the air *prana (life-force)*, provides our primary sustenance. Prana is the life-giving element that we get from the air. So, the more prana you breathe in, the more alive you are and the more you extend your life.

Yogis believe that life-force is available in all forms of nourishment. They believe that people who do not breathe deeply and partake of this life-force from the air suffer from nervous, diseased and weakened bodies and shorter lives.

Think of movement as your life extender, because that is what it is. Exercise seems a small price to pay for vitality and a longer, richer life. Yoga and dance are fun exercises.

Yoga is a simple, relaxed breathing and stretching. Stand with your feet apart and comfortable. Empty all the air from your lungs by slowly exhaling through your nose at the same time that you contract (suck in) your abdomen as far as possible. Now very slowly inhale through your nose at the same time that you push out your abdominal muscles. Hold briefly, about eight seconds, and let out slowly.

This breathing should be very comfortable. Repeat until a sense of ecstasy is attained, holding your breath longer as you get good at it. Yogis recommend that you focus on the stretch and the magic that the stretching does.

As you breathe in, start stretching by raising your arms slowly and relaxedly towards the sky. Stretch, reaching for the ceiling with your fingers. Hold your breath as you breathe in and stretch comfortably. Breathe out as you let the stretch out.

It is not necessary to go immediately to the next stretch. Take a moment to get your breath. Yoga should be done in a relaxed manner. If you want to hold a stretch through two or three deep breaths, that is fine also. Then go on to the next stretch.

Photobiotics

Did you ever wonder why sitting in the sun feels so good? We are incapable of existing without light. Using light correctly can restore the body's electromagnetic framework. Photobiotics is based on the premise that our bodily functions are impossible without light and color. Light (fire), air and water contain a basic nutrient, electrical energy, which gives life. All matter is considered condensed light. If you have health, then you are spectrally balanced, and if you are ill, you are spectrally unbalanced.

Tai Chi & Qi Dong

Reduces some stress hormones, helps joint disorders, heart disease, high blood pressure substance abuse and stress, delays decline of the cardiovascular system and is even safe for those with arthritis. It reduces the risk of falling by profoundly grounding a person, improves consciousness, reduces pain, increases energy, improves concentration, has the same effect as brisk walking, increases strength, strengthens immune system and oxygenates the body.

Yoga or exercise in any of the forms we have been discussing will be your source of energy so you will want to be faithful to it. The new requirements for exercise state that it needs to be done a minimum of thirty minutes everyday to maintain good health.

Start slowly and work up to it. Research has shown that cross training, doing a variety of exercises is best. For example, I run everyday, do Yoga and isometric exercises and do dancing as therapy to help free my soul and spirit.

Dance Therapy

Psychological stress, tension and anguish can be relieved by simply giving your body the attention it needs to relax. One of the more potent ways of doing this is dance therapy. It boosts your mood and mind and promotes a deep sense of well-being. It is a good way especially for artistic people to express themselves and constructively let out feelings and emotions that otherwise would be left inside.

Dance offers mind-body healing much like Yoga in that a re-balancing occurs at the same time that the body is conditioned. Through dance one is able to relax while freeing the mind and body of stress and tension. It enables participants to become more aware of their feelings and discover things about themselves through expressing them.

Dance can be an illuminating experience if practiced on a regular basis. It is especially good for those who are shy, self-conscious and uncomfortable in their bodies. It promotes sleep, weight loss and helps relationships because of the way it relaxes and gets people in touch with themselves. It can be a valuable tool for lifting depression. In fact, dance therapy has been successful in lifting depressions that drugs failed to lift. That is because humans are designed to move, for movement brings us relief. Energy and creativity are liberated when angry feelings and anxiety are expressed.

Even people who exercise for five minutes twice a day experience tremendous benefits as well. In fact, if you are one of those people who don't have "time" to exercise the minimum thirty minutes everyday, there are some simple Yoga exercises that you can do for just five minutes twice a day at your desk that will extend your life and its quality considerably. You can dance in your room for five minutes a day and receive great health benefits. Don't believe me? Well, this is your opportunity to prove something to yourself. Anyway, research has proved:

Exercise, A Little Bit'll Do You

"Studies point to inactivity as a major contributing cause of chronic illnesses. Those who don't exercise face nearly twice the risk for developing heart disease as those who work out regularly"[90]

Exercise Is The Fountain Of Youth

"Recent studies in physiology show that exercise by the middle aged and elderly can turn back the clock 10 to 25 years."[91]

CAN EXERCISE FIGHT THE EFFECTS OF AGING?

"Most of what we think about aging is wrong," said California physician Walter Bortz II, former president of the American Geriatrics Society. "Most declines people consider inevitable are actually a result of disuse."[92]

Walking Found To Aid Heart, Regardless Of Pace[93]

MODERATE WORKOUTS REDUCE STRESS,

---

[90]   © 1993 by The Washington Post, Washington, D.C. Reprinted with permission.

[91]   © 1986 by The New York Times Company. Reprinted by permission.

[92]   © 1991 by The New York Times Company. Reprinted by permission.

[93]   © 1991 by The New York Times Company. Reprinted by permission.

ANXIETY, DEPRESSION[94]

De-Stress Yourself
"Regular Exercise Helps Maintain Health Under Pressure"[95]

The Exercise Rx
"No depression can stand up to a 10-mile run."[96]

LOSS OF IRON LINKED TO EXERCISE
"The best way to help offset the loss of iron caused by exercise is by eating a variety of iron-rich foods..."[97]

If you do the Yoga exercises included here twice a day for five minutes at your desk you will experience a profound improvement in the pain in your back, neck and shoulders. Depressed? As you now know, no depression can endure if you exercise three to four times a week faithfully, and look at all the choices of exercises you have to choose from. And make it fun!

Depression cannot exist if you follow the advice in this book. It is a state that people feel it is okay to sink into because of a series of disasters that have happened to them.

Balance is important to health and mental clarity and keeping the body functioning in optimal condition. Yoga and dance are perfect for this, because both balance. Balance is important for if the mental, physical or spiritual are even

---

[94]   © 1993 by The Washington Post, Washington, D.C. Reprinted with permission.

[95]   © 1993 by The Washington Post, Washington, D.C. Reprinted with permission.

[96]   © 1990 by The Washington Post, Washington, D.C. Reprinted with permission.

[97]   © 1993 by The Washington Post, Washington, D.C. Reprinted with permission.

slightly off, health can become impaired. It is common knowledge now that exercise helps the body heal, rejuvenate and revitalize itself as it increases the flow of blood and the amount of oxygen in it.

Exercise is a fountain of youth all by itself. Your stiffness and soreness will gradually disappear as you exercise, for your body will become more toned, and as the pain goes away, your consciousness will increase. The pains and burdens of life will seem less heavy. You'll be getting a lot in return for even a five or ten minute investment per day. Of course you are encouraged to go for thirty minutes.

The Aging Brain: The Mind Is Resilient, It's The Body That Fails

"Study suggests disease underlies most mental declines."[98]

The Benefits of PQQ, notoriously known for restoring the brain

PQQ stands for pyrroloquinoline quinone. This compound was identified as an essential nutritional component in 1994. Eventually, it will be classified as a vitamin. It's particularly important for the health of the mitochondria. "It appears that PQQ is really the spark of life," Murray says. "Our mitochondria definitely require this compound to produce energy. It's also critical in protecting the mitochondria from damage." The number of catalytic conversions that PQQ can be utilized for is in the realm of over 20,000 times. No other vitamin does that.

---

[98]   © 1991 by The New York Times Company. Reprinted by permission.

Chapter 25

> # MIND AND BODY,
> # ARE THEY ONE?

Increasingly, research indicates that they are. The nervous system and the immune system are linked. The same chemicals that control our moods also control tissue integrity. Therefore, emotions are one of the keys to health. When Freud said the mind creates diseases and it can cure them people called him crazy.

Yet now, fifty-five years after his death, research confirms his statement. Examine the fact that an allergy sufferer can look at a picture of a flower and begin to sneeze, that a hypnotic suggestion can cause a burn on a person's skin, and you can see the power of mind over body. Because what really caused these things are the peoples' minds.

Since bodily functions are controlled by thought and thoughts can mobilize killer cells as well as healing endorphins, we can see the direct connection between the brain and the immune system. Stress also suppresses immune response, another mind-body connection.

Freud said neurosis takes the form of disease, and that emotional turmoil and repressing emotions can produce illness. I checked this out on myself, and found, over and over, that it's true. Every time I have some emotional trauma in my life, I get sick a few days later. I'll bet if you take notice you will find the same to be true about you too.

Having read literally hundreds of articles about cases of people healing themselves and how faith, beliefs, positive energy and affirmations can accomplish this, I now sometimes chant to myself, "I am strong! I am invincible!" I don't get sick nearly as much as I used to! When I eat, I imagine my food is super-nutritious and strengthening me (actually, it is, but this thinking intensifies the effect). This kind of imagery works! Cancer patients who were told to imagine killer cells in their bodies had more killer cells than those who did not do the imaging.

PLEASE NOTE: *Visualization therapy is not something you put in your head and forget about, it must be done actively, or it does not work.* Something I do almost everyday is get in the sun and imagine myself at the bottom of a billowing whirlwind of healing sunshine and that this sunshine has special healing powers. I close my eyes and imagine it whirling around and through me, and healing every cell. I imagine it penetrating through my skin and I can actually feel its purifying warmth. Yes, this works very effectively! Try it!

I mentioned the man, Norman Cousins who was told he would die, that there was no hope for him to live. Remember the one who checked himself out of the hospital and rented a bunch of comedies? His hope and faith had a lot to do with his cure.

Laughter has an immediate effect on our immune systems, but in order to reap the benefits of this healing, we need to do it on a regular basis. Studies have shown that patients who were shown comedies before surgery healed faster than those that were not.

Angry, cynical people are five times more likely to die before the age of fifty than calm trusting ones. And anger has been shown to damage the heart and blood vessels. Many heart specialists agree that heart disease begins in the mind.

Positive thinking will go a long way in keeping you healthy. Just don't allow the negative things to take precedence. Allow yourself to laugh since laughter releases anxiety, fear, hostility and anger and boosts the immune system. Recognize automatic pessimistic thoughts and argue yourself out of them. If someone is repeatedly getting on your nerves, talk to them about it in a diplomatic manner.

Fall in love. Being in love boosts the immune system and increases longevity. Hope has become known as one of the keys to longevity also. Remember, there is an important lesson to be learned in every conflict. Don't let them get you down. You do have a choice between letting conflicts get you down, or using them to learn the important lessons about life that they teach.

Make this piece of information stick in your mind: if the mind can cause an illness, then certainly it can cure one. Monitor cynical and negative thoughts and weed them out. Sometimes our thoughts can go totally wild when we speculate about others' motives and reasons for things.

Talk to your friends and family, people that are close to you, about what is bothering you. Keeping it in bottles it up! Talking is a cure. As you talk, pent up tension is released and the solution to your problem will come to you. Illness often occurs as a result of pent up anger, emotions and frustration.

We do not need to act and think like each other. Instead, we need to adopt a policy of accepting the differences in each other, for each of us is entitled to our own opinion, whether or not it is right or wrong. Concentrate on the things that do jibe. Realize that the whole relationship is more important than the little parts of it that do not work. Remember, whenever there is a lot of anxiety between two people, there begins to be a need to control. Practice trusting. Learn to forgive.

One of the most important reasons relationships fail is because people miscommunicate and thus, become disillusioned with each other. Then the partners build up defenses against one another and withdraw parts of themselves from the relationship. They become involved with other activities or people to fill this walled-off part of themselves.

One of the most efficient ways of healing is just to visually imagine yourself whole and healed, *perfect*. Since what you think about expands, thinking about yourself as whole, healed and *perfect* sets off a string of endorphins that heal. Stop a moment right now. Sit back. Take some deep breaths and visually imagine yourself whole and healed. Press on the third eye point between your eyes as you take deep breaths and imagine yourself perfect.

The more graphic you can get the better. Mentally go into any hurting areas and imagine the tissues pink and healthy and healed. Feel the power of this imagery as your pain goes away! It may take two minutes of concentrating before you feel a bit of warmth in the area you are trying to heal. It really involves concentrating. Yet it really works! And concentrating like this is an excellent way to boost your brain power.

Imagine yourself perfect, complete, with healthy immune system, skin, bones and teeth and be grateful that you do not need a kidney, liver, or heart transplant and do not have AIDS or cancer. Thirty thousand people in America are waiting for organ transplants.

Think of all the good things you have going in your life. Minimize the bad. Shrink it and throw it far away. Do this whenever you feel stressed or overwhelmed. Thinking of the fact that you don't need an organ transplant, or have AIDS or cancer or something else terrible should certainly help minimize your problems.

You have the power to make anything go away that you want to go away. You have the power to make yourself feel whole and at peace. Life is pretty wonderful after all. We just have to allow it to be so.

Don't ever think of yourself from the point of your faults anymore. Accept you unconditionally, and allow yourself to make mistakes sometimes, and forgive yourself when you do.

Ever read **The Interpretation Of Dreams** by Sigmund Freud? This is your chance to completely psychoanalyze yourself, for free. The book is much more than an interpretation of dreams, it is a complete psychoanalysis of the individual. Keep in mind the Victorian period that it was written in as you discover the truths. You can get it free at the library and you will never have so much fun or enlightenment from any other book!

I have been running for more than twenty-five years. Once or twice on my way back, as I was cooling down, I got in touch with my life-force. The first time this happened it was awesome for me. It was like being in touch with that part of me that had been left over after I died when I had gone into shock. My body was spread out on the hospital bed; but I was not in it. What was left of me, what I believe now was my life-force, had become a part of the light and peacefully watched the team of doctors and nurses who were trying to revive me.

At that time, I could read everyone's mind in the room. It felt as if I knew everything there was to know. At the same time I feel that I had incredible benevolent powers. I was a part of the light and it was a very safe, uplifting, comfortable place. I don't think I have felt that peaceful before or since.

My life-force sort of feels like another person there with me, a protective person who loves and cares about me. It is a force, and it is powerful. That night of death was the first time I ever got in touch with mine. Try and get in touch with yours after strenuous exercise or during meditation. It is a comforting friend.

"Homeopaths conceptualize a "life-force" or "vital force," which they describe as the inherent, underlying, interconnective, self-healing process of the organism. This bioenergetic force is similar to what the Chinese call "chi," the Japanese call "ki," Yogis call "prana," Russian scientists call "bioplasm" and Star Wars characters call "The Force." Homeopaths theorize that this bioenergetic process is sensitive to the submolecular homeopathic medicines. The resonance of the microdose is thought to affect the resonance of the person's life-force."

Reprinted with permission of Dana Ullman, from **Discovering Homeopathy**, published by North Atlantic Books, Berkeley CA. 1991. pg. 15.

Needless to say, I think homeopathic medicines have helped me get in closer touch with my life-force.

We know now that our cells are controlled by what we think. In fact, our minds can change every cell in our bodies. It is so ridiculous that we ever thought we could separate the mind from the body.

People have been able to alter their breast size, heal allergies and skin diseases by using their minds to heal themselves, proving that we do have control over our systems if we would just activate this power. As long as we believe it is not there, it remains dormant.

One of the subjects who healed herself had been suffering unbearably with allergies for 12 years. Yet she was able to stop them cold when told to imagine herself well and free of them.

There have also been studies done with the TB test in which subjects' results came out negative or positive, depending on the directions that were given to them by the administrators of the test rather than what their true reading should have been.

> We must get into the flow of our own yin-yang[99] balance, for it controls the flow of our life stream. It is the flow of this energy that influences the effectiveness of our immune systems. Positive and negative energy have their own influences which affect everything from cellular function to heart rate.

Look around you at all the technology and sophisticated gadgetry of our modern society. If humans can be that innovative using just 10-15 percent of our brains, imagine what we will accomplish as our brains evolve and become increasingly more complex.

I think there will be no limit to what can be accomplished, but the greatest drawback to achieving this unlimited state is our putting limitations on what we can accomplish.

Life is wonderful and beautiful if we could just be grateful and appreciate what we have. On the other hand, there is the down side that we all pretend is not there. We all endure it in cynical, hard-pressed, rude, crude or obnoxious, uptight people that we encounter day to day.

Actually, what you have to think about them is that they are doing themselves in and focus on the nice people you encounter. If you can, be compassionate and benevolent and enlighten them on the harm they are doing to themselves by harboring hostility.

Explain to them that when they feel hatred, cynicism and anger their bodies make harmful hormones, including testosterone, epinephrine and the aggression hormone cortisol, which suppress the immune system. Give them On Aggression by Konrad Lorentz with selected sections highlighted or tabbed and they will not want to be associated with aggression when they find out how primitive it is.

It can be even more helpful if you can supply them with additional hard information like the book by Dr. Redford Williams, The Trusting Heart, with

---

[99]   In Chinese philosophy, yin is the female element that stands for darkness, cold and death. Yang is the male element, source of life and heat.

selected sections highlighted or tabbed. Dr. Williams explains this phenomenon much better than anyone else. Imagine the difference it would make in the world if each person took it upon herself to save another person from hostility in this way. Many experts agree on the following points:

Cynicism And Mistrust
Tied To Early Death

"Angry, cynical people are five times as likely to die under 50 as people who are calm and trusting, a psychiatrist has found."[100]

Study Documents How Anger
Can Impair Heart Function

". . .the study is the first to document a change in heart function brought on by anger; it showed that the heart's pumping efficiency is reduced when people get mad."[101]

Hope Emerges As Key To Success
In Life

"Psychologists are finding that hope plays a surprisingly potent role in giving people a measurable advantage in realms as diverse as academic achievement, bearing up in onerous jobs and coping with tragic illness."[102]

The Secret Of Long Life?
Be Dour And Dependable[103]

---

[100] © 1989 by The New York Times Company. Reprinted by permission.

[101] © 1992 by The New York Times Company. Reprinted by permission.

[102] © 1991 by The New York Times Company. Reprinted by permission.

Chapter 26

AWARENESS, THE DIFFERENCE THAT MAKES ALL THE DIFFERENCE

There are some vital facts that you need to know in order to experience ecstasy in your life on a minute-to-minute hour-to-hour, day-to-day basis. In order to get to the true reality, it is necessary to get away from the petty trivialities of life which can mount and obscure our vision.

In addition to obscuring our vision, petty trivialities like the ones encountered in the work place from day to day can raise blood pressure, increase heart rate, increase adrenaline levels and stomach acids and cause toxins to be released into the body because of the stress. Petty trivialities can be much more than trivial.

In some cases they can be life threatening. Two examples: sexual harassment and emotional harassment. Emotional harassment is the boss popping gum when she knows some of her workers cannot stand it. Both scenarios can make someone a nervous wreck. Stress and nervousness can wreak havoc on bodily functions.

The way our work places in America are set up leads to social isolation since the people that you are dealing with intimately on a day-to-day basis have to be dealt with on a totally superficial level to maintain a professional relationship.

That faulty ideology has been around for so long, it may be that it has led to the alienation and man's humiliation to man that dominates our society more than the loss of the family, small towns and religion. Certainly if people who work together could become more intimate, some of our society's loneliness and despair would be eliminated.

What more convenient place to have a family than in the work place where you spend 40 hours of the week with people? Whether you admit it to yourself or not, the people you work with become intimates because they discover private and personal things about you. It is crazy not to take advantage of this wonderful opportunity to connect with others of our own kind since human relationships are the main treasure of life. Any people you spend 40 or 50 hours of the week with become intimates. It was only because whites got to be around blacks that they realized they are not very different from each other.

When people met socially for church events that extended to everything from baseball leagues to potluck dinners to neighbors looking out for each other to church members preparing food for your wedding or looking after your dying grandmother, there was not nearly so much social isolation, loneliness or crime in our society, for the criminal did not want his peers to disdain him.

Just look back at the fifties; almost every city was a small hometown. Now individuals are lost in cities, drowning in loneliness and isolation, groping aimlessly to connect and spending 50 percent of their lives with people they are told they must only marginally connect with.

No wonder some individuals in our society are confused and frustrated. This behavior is not natural. We humans are in need of each other, but do not know how to connect.

Some people are afraid of letting others know how they really are for fear that they will not be accepted that they simply hide their real selves. They think the difference in them is too great for anyone else to understand. However, if you think about it, we here in America are encased in a culture that exposes us to certain influences, and since we cannot escape these influences it is impossible that we could be that much more different than each other.

Our neighbors are not that much different than we are. If we look at each other with open minds and forget about all the many bad experiences that we have had with other people, and go at building relationships from scratch, based on trust, we may be able to see the quality of our relationships changing because of the change in us.

Getting back to our vision of experiencing ecstasy on a moment-to-moment basis, in order to really focus clearly on what we want, so we can then focus on getting it, we need to relieve our minds of emotional stress and pent up garbage from past traumatic events.

You say you don't have any? That is exactly what I said when a dear friend told me about getting on the true level of reality. I said quickly that there was no one more into awareness and consciousness than I and that I was on the true level of reality more than he or anyone else I knew.

He argued with me, and insisted that I needed to take this basic awareness training that he claimed would put me on the "true level of reality and teach me to live a life I loved and love the life I lived and free me from past traumas and limiting beliefs." "Past traumas?" I said, "I resolved those a long time ago. Limiting beliefs? Why, I studied a lot of philosophy, so my beliefs are right up there with the greats like Socrates, Descartes, Kant, Schopenhauer, Heidegger, Hegel, and Wagner." Just come, he said, you'll find the new awareness invaluable.

Yet many people who say they have no past traumatic events are walking around with a mind-set that someone else out there is going to try to rip them off like some other person did last year, or 10 years ago. The rip-off could be emotional or physical. So they are constantly on their guard about getting ripped off again.

And guess what? Because they are constantly on their guard about being ripped off, they get ripped off. It can be a self-fulfilling prophesy. How much sense does it make for us to expect that every person we meet will try to rip us off?

My fifth response to his persistence that I take the awareness class? I don't need any more awareness, since I am the most aware person I know, I already live a life I love and I don't have any unresolved past traumas. But he would not give up on me and thank goodness he didn't. Finally, he agreed to pay for the training for me on the condition that I would agree to pay him back if I thought it was worth the money.

After much coercing (he actually nearly hounded me to death), and he finally talked my husband into it after he agreed to pay for it for both of us ($450 each) with the agreement that if we did not think the training was worth it we would not have to repay his money, I took the training, thinking, "What makes you think you have three days to devote to deeper awareness when you are already supremely aware? You don't need this."

Yet when I got in the training, I felt very lucky that he had not given up on me and scared that he might have. In the Lifespring Basic Awareness training I found valuable tools that transformed and enriched me powerfully and profoundly. It causes someone who is already having a wonderful life to experience 200 percent more joy and ecstasy in their life.

It had everything my friend promised me, and more! It was awesomely enlightening. With all my education, and my constantly reading, learning and growing, I discovered I really was not exactly living the life I loved. But this awareness training put me on the road to it. To give you some idea of its power, I had six books trapped inside me when I took it, and it was a powerful catalyst that helped me to get them all out.

I had so many breakthroughs that enabled me to understand and see the hurtful aspects of people and things I had dealt with in the past differently, and clearer. Some things I had been sure I had dealt with and overcome were incomplete and I completed them.

I resolved so many of the hurtful events of my past, and experienced such a rapid burst of cognitive growth that I felt high at the end of the training. I stopped living as if my past determined my future and designed the future I wanted. So can you.

Think about this: if you have not done it in 20 or 30 or 50 years, don't think the magic answer is going to come to you. You need help in getting it, and this training is where you can get all the help to get anything in the world that you want, and end up with it (what you want, I mean)!

One example I would like to share is this: years earlier I had discovered that my husband was having an affair with my best friend. At the time I said to myself, I am not going to allow this to hurt me, I am not going to permit either of those slimeballs get me upset.

I thought they can slink on off under the carpeting and rot somewhere, because as far as I was concerned, that was how I left them. I left him and started divorce proceedings, cut myself off from both of them and found and married my second husband. I did not even think about them for years.

Fifteen years later I have this training and I get in touch with how deeply I had been hurt, and how I had stuffed the hurt somewhere deep inside myself, determined never to see or feel it, yet I had in fact been carrying it around all those years.

That was one of the more painful purges, but during the training, I encountered at least ten other unresolved traumas that I had completely forgotten, or was it that I blocked them out, thinking I had resolved them and dealt with them when I had not completely? Many seemed insignificant, like an incident with my sister at age six, but I found it had a profound, deeper meaning.

I cried for one solid week. At the end of that time I felt ten pounds lighter, I felt emotionally free. I felt exhilarated, and I realized for the first time how heavy that garbage had been to carry around. One of the more remarkable things was that my lower back, which had been sore for a long time, suddenly had no pain in it!

Along with the other people in the training, I had numerous such breakthroughs which enabled me to stop living as if my past was me, or had everything to do with me, and enabled me to plot and plan my life the way I wanted it to be from then on, leaving the past behind, and resolved. Unbelievably, people go around with this story about themselves from their past that has nothing to do with who they are today. I realized I had made up a story about myself to myself that was just that, a story, and not really me.

This is all much more powerful than it sounds, and in order to be fully appreciated, must be experienced, and I challenge you to do it. If you are not exceptionally pleased with the training, please feel free to write me, although I am sure you will write to praise this training which allows us to dynamite away our perimeters and really live and attain what we really want in life and be free to be completely happy.

People who had known me a long time asked me, "What have you done to yourself, you're different?" I'll say I was different! I was transformed. These were my friends, but when I tried to tell them what had transformed me, it was hard to communicate it because this phenomenal mode of cognitive growth needs to be experienced.

Therapy doesn't always get rid of these kinds of things, and we can't get rid of them by ourselves. If that were possible, we would have done it by now. What is needed is participation in a self-actualization group, like **Lifespring's Basic Awareness Training,** (phone 301-951-0090 in the Washington, DC area. They have offices in most major cities). Another valuable training for improving relationships is **John Gray Seminars** (phone 1-800-821-3033. They are also in most major cities).

I have participated in a dozen or so awareness trainings since then and experienced the most benefit from these two. If you go out and take one now you will be terrified to think that this is something that you might have missed in your life. It will really blow your mind! I can honestly say that it is the single most important thing I have ever done to further develop myself in my entire life.

On a scale of one to ten, comparing this training to college, college is a two and it is a ten. But only those who take it will truly know its value. Just go out and take it right away because they (the Lifespring organization), guarantee that you can have your money back if you don't think the basic awareness training is worth the bargain price,[104] whatever it is, because what you will get from there is priceless.

This is basic reality training and I don't care how much you think you are in the real reality, you aren't until you know what they teach you. You experience dozens of universal truths, which is totally different from reading about them. I guarantee you it is worth a million dollars if you have not done something like it before. I feel very sure that after you do it, you will say that this awareness training is the most important thing you have ever done in your life. And if you do not agree, you can let me know.

Out of 850,000 people only three or four have asked for refunds, and that was because they'd had a similar training. It is an awesomely illuminating experience that everyone needs to experience, for it dynamites away the perimeters of our limitations and accelerates our evolution about 250 percent. If you are stuck in some aspect of your life and/or miserable about some things, no matter what they are, you will find the solution to them either during or soon after you take this training. I guarantee it.

---

[104]   They had a special rate for public service providers like teachers, nurses, doctors, policemen, etc. of $200.

Dr. Albert Ellis, the internationally renowned cognitive psychologist states that anyone who allows herself to be upset or unhappy for more than thirty seconds is cheating herself and wasting good energy and life's precious moments on negative stuff. At a seminar he gave (he is a cognitive genius, and simply brilliant) a woman, clearly beaten by life, shoulders bowed, remorseful expression, got up and said she was afraid since she was going to be working with a man who wrote her up as incompetent in the past when she worked for him that he was going to do the same thing again, which would really hurt her at this company where she was working on a career as she had been there thirteen years. She also implied that maybe she might be a little incompetent but she did not want her company to know that.

Dr. Ellis rebuked her on that. "Just because you are incompetent as a secretary, or let me put it this way, even if you are incompetent as a secretary, that does not diminish your status as a person. Nothing should diminish your status, especially to yourself."

I thought, how wise he is.

Try these strategies:

- If things do not work out as you expected, that does not mean that everything is hopeless. Look instead at all the things that did work out. Suppose all the things that had gone right had gone wrong, and compare the value of that to the value of the one thing going wrong.

- Don't give so much weight to one single defeat. There is the rest of your life to be lived, and many victories to achieve. Taking a single defeat and allowing it to make a fatality of you is a manifestation of low self-esteem. Raise your esteem. You will find that you are worth it.

- Don't dwell on the negative. Many people magnify the negative things in their lives/or about themselves by going over and over them, as if in disbelief that this could happen or be. You are in control of your mind, so control this by beating down negative thoughts and realize they are a pattern that you must break. Instead, relish in the positive. Remember, it outweighs the negative.

- Eliminate "should" statements from your life. Statements like I should own a home by now, or we should be taking a vacation this year, or I should be able to buy that. Instead, participate in your life 100 percent as if each day is the last day of your life. Share yourself with others genuinely. You receive back what you put out in life. Surrender yourself to the ones you love. No risk equals no gain. Experience and feel life now, fully, for this is no dress rehearsal. Stop waiting for some event in the future, like finding your true love, to live fully. Wipe out limiting beliefs and accept the differences in others. Life is experienced through involvement with others.

Don't try to read other peoples minds for very often when we do, we are wrong. Don't conclude about people. You can think that because of a series of events happening that there could be no other possible explanation. Well, very often, there is. Find out the facts before you conclude.

Your problems are no greater than anyone else's. Life is difficult for all of us.

Don't expect people to live up to your recipe of how they are supposed to be or act. Accept people as they are, and you can gain the contribution that others can make to your life. Interfering with them, making them live by your rules distorts how they would have normally interacted with you, and you lose valuable insight that you might have gained.

Don't judge.

The following article **Committed Interaction** is reprinted with permission of **Lifespring**, 4650 East West Highway, Bethesda Maryland 20815, phone 301-951-0090. They have offices in most major cities.

If you want to get an example of the power of improving your life by heightening your awareness, there are some tapes by Wayne Dyer that will give you a good idea of what I am talking about. For even though they are powerful

COMMITTED INTERACTION

By Ann P. Miller

If you could name an area of your life in which you expend the most energy and learn the most, what would it be? If you're not sure, ask yourself which area of your life gives you the most joy—and pain? For many people, the response is relationships. Many students graduate from the Lifespring Basic Training with a renewed sense of the importance of relationships in their lives. Graduates leave the Training with fresh perspectives on their interactions with and their commitment to their mates, their parents, their siblings, their friends, their co-workers.

What do graduates do with that fresh perspective? What in their lives is informed by their experience of a renewed commitment to fuller, richer relationships? These are not new questions for most of us, who've described our experiences of the Lifespring trainings to others.

I wanted to hear what graduates had to say about their primary relationships after the Training. Yet, like love, peace, and happiness, working relationships can be difficult to discuss.

But when a relationship isn't working, there is usually something concrete to discuss. In fact, we often don't discover, or at least face, the truth about a relationship until we are in a crisis or break-down about it. So in talking to graduates, I framed my questions in the context of breakdown.

Consider the experience of crisis or breakdown in your relationships. What happens for you when an unpredictable event or situation occurs which stops the forward motion of the relationship? Do you avoid your partner, confront him or her, or maintain 'normal' condi-

tions despite the upset? What conditions determine breakdown in your relationships? Lack of communication, or lack of agreement on certain issues, even absence? It takes two to make a relationship, but only one to make an illusion. A breakdown is no small event, no minor squabble or disagreement, but rather a fundamental point of disjuncture between two people's experience in their relationship.

While I was researching this article, I had dinner with a married grad, who asked, "Why is it that people get married?" She and her husband of ten months were having what she called "a stormy week," and she was exhausted from the constant emotional roller-coaster ride. She wondered aloud, "Why does this society believe we should live with someone else all the time?" Listening to her, I heard her core question as a much more personal one. Amid her breakdown with her husband, she was asking herself, "What am I committed to in this marriage? Why am I spending my life with this man?" These moments of complete and fundamental honesty with ourselves can be some of the most significant in the face of our commitment.

In my conversations with graduates around the country, I noticed that in every response, these people held their primary relationships as a partnership, as a shared commitment they work together to accomplish. As one graduate put it, "There are no percentages of

participation that make up a relationship that works. We are partners, and everything comes out of that."

With so much at stake, how partners respond in a breakdown becomes critical. In choosing how we show up, we shape our own interaction and impact, and fundamentally, our own transformation.

> When I ask, from a committed stand on my relationship, 'what do I bring forth here, what am I willing to offer,' I am also asking, 'what can I contribute to this person's life.'

Recognition of the choices we make, particularly when things aren't working, can assist us in moving through crises.

When Kathy and James Black of San Francisco, California, took the Basic together in 1986, they realized their marriage was in breakdown—they felt it had lost its aliveness. "We were very comfortable with each other, with the way things were, so there was no movement or excitement in our relationship. I realized that marriage is a daily commitment, and not something worth having if you're only going through the motions." In losing sight of what they were committed to together, the Blacks had lost interest in vital movement together.

Being willing to have the best of what's there and work out the worst is no simple task. It requires commitment, else we would 'give up on' what's there. It requires engaging a new set of perspectives, actions and possibilities. James and Kathy took the opportunity of breakdown to "realign or redefine

Continued on next page . . .

what it was we were committed to, and we saw that our relationship was worth whatever it took" to fulfill each of them. They realized that they were missing a key aspect of personal and mutual satisfaction, which was "to support each other in enjoying all the things available to us, and expanding ourselves individually through involvement in other activities." By shifting their perspective on their marriage, they built a new structure for mutual satisfaction, and thus for accomplishment.

Asking questions about what I want to keep and what I want to add takes some consideration of how else my commitment can be fulfilled. As our relationships shift and adjust, one partner may be experiencing interruption or breakdown while the other is unaware of or oblivious to their experience, and often not in that process of breakdown.

do I care about here?' And always when I could be honest, it was him, me, us together. I wouldn't give up, which was a shift for me, and he finally saw the value in that. I don't know how it happened, but he shifted. And then our whole relationship moved to a whole other place, another realm of interaction. It was, still is, incredible."

If we hold a caring, productive relationship as a true accomplishment in our lives, facing the questions about our commitment is essential to personal satisfaction. Because when I ask, from a committed stand on my relationship with another, 'what am I bringing forth here, what am I willing to offer, to have between us,' I am also asking 'what can I contribute to this person's life.'

Responding to these questions may illuminate a radically different relationship. And it may end the

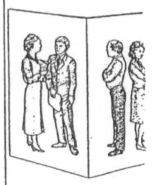

to her husband, and his actions. After the training, "I went to him and said 'I now see my role in this, and I acknowledge that role.' The results of this conversation were that we created a framework for a very caring friendship which continues to expand and enrich our lives and the lives of our two daughters."

Jilly's ex-husband also enrolled in the Basic, and since then their two daughters have participated in Lifespring programs also. "The difference for us now is that we are willing to have love be there in our relationship, which is best expressed as friends. And this new way of being together has opened up multitudes of possibilities for us." Their current situation reflects their willingness to consider where their commitment lies, and to build on that rather than on an outmoded framework.

Several graduates emphasized communication as the key indicator in relationships. As one Maryland woman put it, "the main breakdown in my relationships, including my marriage, is in not hearing what is said. I've learned that if he says he doesn't want to be in a committed relationship, believe him." Beth Blair of Washington, D.C. sees that "not talking about my expectations, not telling the truth—to myself, and to him—is the main thing. When I do tell the truth with him, I'm supporting both of us in the relationship, instead of saying to myself, 'maybe

---

Breakthrough doesn't have to be catharsis; seeing distinctions about how we are enables powerful shifts and often subtle changes.

Charlene and James Parks who live now in Chicago, reached a point in their marriage where, as Charlene puts it, "we realized we weren't in the same relationship. We would have conversations where James would say, 'Yeah everything's fine, we're doing great,' and I'd be shocked. So, I took a deep breath and said, 'No, everything is not great. I'm miserable, and we need to talk through these problems.' But he wouldn't hear that, wouldn't look even at what I saw and felt as problems; he dismissed them with superficial solutions that never worked."

Charlene continued to communicate her experience to her husband, and "finally James began to listen, and to look. And then we could look together, and we did move through that crisis. What it took from me was a constant, plodding patience and honesty about my experience with him. And everytime I found myself losing it, I'd stop and ask myself, 'what

relationship as it exists. Divorce is an end to the partnership of marriage; yet many couples continue as partners in raising their children or in friendship. A relationship continues, but it embodies other commitments than that of marriage.

Jilly Houston of Reston, VA who went through a divorce ten years ago, says that in many relationships, "when we hit a problem, we tend to throw the baby out with the bath water." And when that happens, it is more difficult to learn how to avoid the same situation next time.

When Jilly took the Basic Training, a few years after her divorce, she looked at her role in her marriage. "I became accountable for my role in our relationship, which meant I became accountable for the results. I saw how the only possible result was divorce." In clarifying for herself the difference between blame and accountability, Jilly could look clearly at her actions, her reactions

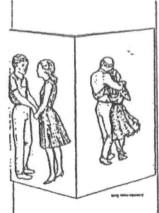

he doesn't want to hear how I feel and what I want." Because once we talk, we can find out if we want different things in the relationship at that point."

Pat Taylor in San Francisco recognizes breakdown in her marriage as "when we are not listening to each other. We get very positioned on who's right, and there are feelings of anger and hurt." When Pam notices this condition, she stops and asks herself, "what's not working, and what would work. If I'm seeing these conditions, I've already moved out of 'breakdown' since it just takes me getting off my ego, and going back to what I care about in the relationship. Then I communicate what I see to him, and listen to him."

In the process of being open to another person, to the myriad interactions among two individuals' concerns, habits, dreams, worries, feelings, and beliefs, we have the opportunity to confront everything that matters to us.

Drew Allen, a lawyer in Hamlin New York, considers breakdown as the condition of his "unwillingness to confront the issue or the other person involved." In that state, he usually gives himself two options. "I withdraw from the situation or the person, or I act as if I'm saying to them, 'go your own way, and the heck with it; I'll do it myself.' Either way, I am getting no feedback, and I am putting negative energy into the relationship with

my fear about dealing with the issue or the person, so the relationship can go quickly bankrupt."

Recognizing what we automatically do in breakdown, and how it does or does not support our commitment in the relationship is the first step toward looking for another way of being about it. I can decide how I will resolve an issue, and act on that resolution, yet still not change my perception of the situation or issue. And it may be my perception, what I am telling myself about the situation, that is limiting my progress in the matter. Once Drew sees the limits of his habitual options, he has shifted his perspective on the situation. Instead of relying on reflexive behavior for protection and security, he can discover another way of being that allows a fulfilling relationship.

In taking a moment to stop, look, and choose how to be now, we step out of the irrelevant framework the past, and our reflexive behavior, has become. If we don't shift our perception of the situation, we will select from what

me. . Paul White of Sterling, Virginia sees his role as a financial services consultant as one in partnership with his clients. In examining those partnerships, he has found that "integrity, the certainty that what I'm doing for my clients conforms to my values of justice and integrity," is his commitment in those relationships. "When I am up against a problem situation, I ask myself, 'is this a question of integrity?'

If it is not a question of integrity, Paul looks at how he is being in the situation, which he sees as a system of interaction. "Breakdown doesn't mean failure. Especially if I start with the premise that all systems can be right, and all systems can be improved. Breakdown is really an opportunity to look at the system of interaction and improve it. From that perspective, it's much easier to let go of what I'm doing, knowing I started with it as 'the best I can think of now' and knowing too that it may be inappropriate in this new situation." Focussed on what matters now, he is free to consider how else the relationship can be.

In being open to another person, . . . we have the opportunity to confront everything that matters to us.

---

we already know. Innovation and creative solutions don't exist in what we already know.

A key source for innovation lies in making distinctions about what is happening and what we are committed to have happen in the relationship. Bill Freeman of Garrison, New York, has learned that "when I stop communicating, and become self-centered about something" it's time to "realize that how I'm being is not how I say I want the relationship to be. So I get over it, and start talking, and clear the air between us." Once the 'air is cleared,' we can begin again. Breakthrough doesn't have to be catharsis; seeing distinctions about how we are enables powerful shifts and often subtle changes.

Once I see each partnership I'm in as integral to my life's accomplishment, I act on what matters to

When we hold crises as interruptions in a satisfying and contributory life, instead of as indictments of failure, we offer ourselves another view. In a conversation that began with the word breakdown, graduates talked about commitment. Within a context of 'what happens when things fall apart' graduates related what held everything together. Every graduate I talked to described their relationship breakdown as a valuable experience, a discovery process, even a lasting lesson. Each of these people found a kernel of truth in the crisis, and gleaned possibility from that truth. From this perspective, they saw innovative and fulfilling solutions. Their conversation about relationships is truly a conversation for possibility!

and transforming, they are about one tenth as powerful as the Lifespring Basic Awareness Training.

The tapes are called **The Awakened Life** (45-59 dollars), available through Nightingale Conant at 1-800-525-9000. They carry a money-back guarantee so if you don't like them, you can send them back and get a refund. I don't think you will, as you will want to share them with the people you love.

The "Other"

Carson McCullers, the author of **The Heart Is A Lonely Hunter** developed a theory of "the other." The other is that which we wish and wait and pine for that we don't have. The irony of the other is that many forego living fully in the moment, for they are waiting to live fully when they get their other. The tragedy is that more often than not, when they get their other, things are not as they imagined they would be, and so, they no longer want it as they had, but replace it immediately, as soon as they attain it, with another other. This results in their not living as fully as they could if it were not for this other that kept them longing for tomorrow, waiting to live fully then. The *Theory of Diminishing Returns* is hard at work here. In it, the greatest satisfaction is gained with the first bite of pizza, and every subsequent bite becomes less delicious. The secret is to be happy with what you have and live and exist happily in each moment, for life and health are precious and meant to be lived fully now. Very often what we have is great, and we can't see the greatness until it's gone, or things change.

About 20 years ago I read a research article about the results of a study of **The Mirror Effect** which is a situation which exists when people judge themselves according to how they see themselves in the mirror. As they age and watch their bodies deteriorate in the mirror, they devalue themselves. This can be especially true of acne sufferers, who can be somewhat scorned by the general un-acned population. You've heard people say, "Oh I was hell in my day, but now the looks are gone; I'm old, I'm bald, I forget things, I can barely get it up..." and what they are saying, in effect, is that their value has diminished along with their body's deterioration.

As Albert Ellis pointed out, no one should measure their value that way. Let's assume that the person speaking who said "Oh I was hell in my day, but now I'm old. . ." is retired and sits home all day watching soap operas and eating potato chips and drinking coffee. For dinner he goes to a cafeteria where he can get a meal inexpensively. This could be nutritious food, but cafeteria food is often out of the can or held on a steam table until most of the essential nutrients are gone.

Since the body is a machine and it performs according to the fuel and maintenance it receives, what do you think the chances are that the man mentioned above is going to be in poor health? Two of the first things to deteriorate when the body is deficient are sexual and mental functioning.

However, if he were a person who had been running and eating fortified and organic foods for years, taking vitamins, acidophilus and oxygen to kill free-radicals, fortifying foods by adding organic tofu[105] to bread and pasta recipes, drinking liquified vegetable and fruit juices two or three times a day, he would not be in poor health. As you know, all of the above will enhance health, for they have powerful healing abilities.

Yet all these things I had been doing for my body did not make my face more attractive. Only Retin-A, the exfoliants I use, and me re-forming my face made that difference.

The implications of what all this means are staggering when you consider how it will add new vigor, lots of more beautiful, intelligent people, and older mothers and fathers to our society.

The effect looking young has had on my life has been incredible. Here's an example: I'm close to fifty, I have two grown children and two grandchildren,

---

[105]   Commercially grown soybeans, which tofu is made of, are sprayed with herbicides and pesticides so heavily that I do not recommend eating them.

one five, and one four. I look like I'm twenty. It was not something I planned but three years ago a young man came to my door selling encyclopedias. We became friends, and within a few months this friendship blossomed into love. He was very mature, extremely well educated and charming. I did not find out until months later that he was only 29 years old. In fact, he conducted himself so that I never even dreamed that he was not my age.

My grown children had a fit, their reason: "Mom, he's too young for you!" But by this time I had no doubt that he was not! Besides, he was more open-minded than men my age and not so set in his ways. And when he told me he felt the same way, there seemed to be no turning back. There wasn't. And we have been very happy and compatible. Should I give up a relationship that feeds my soul just because my children don't approve?

And now he wants to have a child of his own, never having had one, and since studies have shown that healthy older mothers (over forty) most likely have normal children, I may well have one. Since I am in excellent health and physical condition there is no reason why I should not. So you can see what looking younger can present.

That is one of the reasons I recommend the **Lifespring Basic Awareness Training** so that the mental can keep aligned with the physical. It is amazing how these little things like **The Demonstration Effect** and **The Mirror Effect** can creep in without our realizing it. The awareness training minimizes these kinds of things. It balances in a way that nothing else does.

Put all your prejudices aside and just go in and try it. If you don't like what you hear, ask for a refund. Boy will your life ever change for the better if you stay. And if you were good already, you'll be 250 percent better.

Your mental state is the most important aspect of anything, especially looking young. Yet that doesn't work properly if you are not nourishing your body correctly. Your looks and health can be seriously affected. As you know, even slight imbalances and deficiencies in our bodies' chemical systems can have enormous effects.

Haven't you seen people in their twenties who acted as if they were in their forties? This is usually a result of a past condition or environment, like being brought up in an old-fashioned environment. As you live day-to-day and learn and grow, you take yourself out of that mind-set. Our entire lives are lived as a mental and physical experience inside our heads. And we can make ourselves miserable or happy, just by the thoughts that we allow ourselves to have.

Which brings us to another important topic, how do you treat yourself? You have the power, you know, to be good to yourself and remain calm and relaxed and feeling ecstasy all the time, and you also have the power to make your life miserable, to worry and fret and dwell on the negative, be afraid, aggressive, cynical, etc. If you stop and think about it, your life is exactly what you have made out of it so far. You are having the kind of life that you designed for yourself. You are making the salary that you feel you deserve, living in the kind of house you feel you deserve. How do you like it?

You probably treat yourself the way you know you should be treated. Think about that question. Do you? For me it means trying to enjoy every moment of my life and appreciating the profound specialness of my time here on earth. Do extra special things for yourself sometimes. You know what I mean as we all have our favorites. Mine is going for long walks on beautiful sunny days or working outside, or just being outside. I love to sneak away sometimes and see a matinee in the middle of the week when everyone else is working and I am supposed to be working too.

Sometimes we just deserve a reward for hanging in there and doing the right things. Did you get so busy trying to survive that you forgot to give yourself some fun and relaxation every now and then? You can gage this by how much you laugh every week. Keep a tally in your head of how much you laugh for a month. If this is no dress rehearsal, when are you going to have enough joy and laughter in your life? Are you unconsciously waiting for a time to have it? you should be having joy and ecstasy every minute right now.

Recent research has proved that the kinds of hormones and endorphins our bodies create when we feel joy and sadness, cynicism and anger are different. And the winners for most destructive are cynicism and anger.

How much quality time do you spend with the ones you love? How close are your close friends? Are they what you want them to be? Are you pretending some things about your friendships and relationships that you are not being fully honest with yourself about? How much do you really trust your best friend, close relative, husband? Do you have a consistent pattern of failure or success in relationships?

How do your friends and family see you? If you really look at it and stop pretending some things, can you honestly say you are happy with your relationships? Do the people who know you see you as you see yourself? The awareness training will address all these issues for you and you will experience a profound new sense of yourself and how to get on the track you want to be on in your life and in your relationships.

Can it be possible that you have gotten yourself into a mode of rushing from one activity to the other, rushing the hours of the day, the minutes of your life, by? I call a Type-A person who rushes through the events of their life, whether consciously or unconsciously, rushing is at the back of everything that person does. Many people get themselves into a mode of rushing the hours of the day by so that the workday can be over with. There is no reason why people cannot enjoy being at work.

They think that when they get home and relax that they are going to be fine. Only when they get home and try to relax, they can't because they have put themselves into a mode of rushing, and once it's turned on, it's hard to turn off. Yes, you guessed it, the awareness training will help you turn it off.

Unfortunately, when one puts oneself into a mode of rushing the hours by, the rushing does not automatically stop when the workday is over. Once in the rush mode, people, without even realizing it, rush through their lives the same way they mentally rush those hours of the clock away at the office all day. It's like living in a wind tunnel. In order to stop this eternal rushing and begin enjoying life again we have to turn the wind off, which means we have to force our lives to slow down.

To slow down we can take a break and reassess and start again with new plans and priorities. There are several escapes from your hectic life that you can plan that are not just affordable, but are true escapes! One of them is the three day Lifespring Basic Awareness Training. A trip to the beach, or to Paris won't give you what you'll get there: peace of mind, contentment, resolution of your problems. Doing all those things will make you high!

Another solution for temporary escape from the rat race - - **get a massage,** get involved in a sport, take a class or workshop or take time for something you like to do. Take responsibility for getting enough relaxation, play and fun.

If, upon examination, you find you are not being as good to yourself as you should be, and are finding yourself frustrated and angry a lot, if you are putting your needs second to those of anyone else's, or continuing in an abusive relationship, or putting living on hold until something happens in the future, which doesn't exist yet, then you need to stop right this moment and figure out what you need to do to put your needs first and put you here in the present because the present is your life and your life should not be lived waiting for something in the future. Now is the only time of your life!

You need to ask yourself, as you answer the above questions, how it came to be that you are living for when, instead of NOW?!

Now is the only reality, and perhaps we think this way because of some of the great existentialists, like Descartes, Sartre, Kierkegaard, Hegel, and Heidegger, to name a few. Get yourself grounded in it, for they were right. Savor life and stop waiting to live fully. Live fully right **now!** Suppose you had been one of those discharged sperm that did not make it to the egg? Suppose your mother had aborted you? Just thinking about these facts should help you to make every moment of your life a celebration.

This entire world exists according to words and concepts that humans made up. When you think about that, it is pretty profound. I mean, there really is no such thing as time, or space, or beauty. These are merely words for concepts that we coined as those concepts.

People who know they can do it have the ability to change their lives and destinys. Everyone's success depends on how they see life, and how much success they think they can get. Usually, it has been proved to be true that people can only be as successful as they think they can be. Thought can be one of the most powerful things on earth, for it begets action.

Back to the movie, **Field Of Dreams**? Disasters were happening in the midst of fantastic miracles. It turned out that all the people had to do was do the best they could and "go the limit" and trust, and it all worked out beautifully. Life is like that too. We just have to make that choice about being positive and happy and stick with it.

The following books changed my life profoundly. I think they will change your life also. They are: **Unlimited Power** by Anthony Robbins, **The Road Less Traveled** by Scott Peck, **Introduction To Modern Existentialism** by Ernst Breisach.

Chapter 27

HEAL THE HEART,
FEED THE SOUL

When you resolve past conflicts in the way that they will be resolved when you do one of the trainings mentioned in the last chapter, you will be healing your heart and feeding your soul. You, in essence, become whole.

One thing that has always interested me is the question, what is the meaning of life? Taking awareness trainings has helped bring me closer to finding out the meaning of life. Have you already found the answer? I will tell you later what I have discovered the meaning of life to be.

Some other things that heal the heart and feed the soul:

Sunshine

Laughter

Knowledge

Kisses

Hugs. Research has proved that hugs are beneficial to health. Human beings need love and affection. In addition, they need loving, caring, caressing, cuddling and snuggling.

Joy. Whatever brings you joy also produces healing endorphins in your body.

Being with someone you love. Especially your lover. Even if its not a lover, but a friend, or a baby you love. We heal our hearts and receive nourishment for our souls in our relationships with the people we love. Caution on love: Plato said we believe others think as we do, so usually when we accuse someone of something, that thing is true about us.

Being outside on a beautiful sunshiny day in a beautiful flower garden or outdoor area. Being there with someone you love doubles the fun.

Listening to beautiful music.

Looking at something beautiful everyday, even if it is only the sky.

Experiencing the pheromones of the one you love. These are sexual excitants produced by the apocrine glands. The chemicals in scents of perspiration, saliva, vaginal secretions and urine contain pheromones which affect reproductive and sexual arousal. The most likely reason that people fall in love is these pheromones in the groin area and underarm, even though most people are totally unaware of this fact. Men and women who are around each other experience higher levels of balanced hormones because of the exposure to each other's pheromones.

Attaining a goal

Being in love

Making love

Being told you're beautiful by the one
you love.

Getting a massage.

Meditating. Next time you're beginning to feed your soul by meditating put on some of your favorite music and your favorite scent and this will send your endorphins soaring. Get in your most comfortable position. Empty all the air from your lungs by slowly exhaling through your nose at the same time that you contract (suck in) your abdomen as far as possible. Now very slowly inhale through your nose at the same time that you push out your abdominal muscles. Hold briefly, about eight seconds, and let out slowly. This should be very comfortable. Repeat until a sense of ecstasy is attained, holding your breath longer as you get good at it. Yogis recommend that you focus on the breath and the magic that the breathing does. Many people chant or focus on one point or thing, but I prefer to let my mind run amuck into the farthest reaches of the universe if it wants to at this time. I allow it to go or rest, as it wishes.

Come to peace with life. Come to realize that every disaster has an important lesson to teach us, and that growth occurs through conflict. It is a part of life. As they said in the olden days- we need to trust. Put forth your best effort and never allow obstacles to stand in your way, but see them as stepping stones. As you may have looked around and noticed, all of us are having a hard time at life because that is how life is- difficult. The best way to deal with the fact that life is difficult is to just accept this fact, expect the crap that's forever happening, and learn to look for the important lesson that you needed to learn from the conflict.

I promised to tell you what I have come to think is the meaning of life. Life has no meaning. We give our lives meaning by having goodness, ideals, dreams and goals and people we love. Since our lives are lived entirely in our heads, we have an array of meanings we can give for our lives. Life is meant to be enjoyed moment by moment, and is immensely enhanced by knowledge and growth. We have the capacity to increase our cognitive and intellectual abilities so that our lives feel like a work of art in progress. The most important thing in life? Human relationships.

Come to peace with death. We need to come to realize that matter can not be created or destroyed, it simply goes into different states. We have to die while we are alive to be reborn.[106] What you need to know about death is this: you had a life before you became a fetus, as a sperm and as an egg. Those lives ended when the egg became fertilized and another began. You had a life for nine months as a fetus, and it ended, and you began another as an infant. You had a life as an infant, do you remember it? In each case of a life ending, the past life was never remembered. You are matter going through different states. Even though you have no memory of these lives, you know you had them. So each time you die, you begin a new life in another form, as something else. Having died once, I can tell you that it's not so bad. In fact, it was a pleasant experience.

Come to love ourselves unconditionally. Come to forgive yourself for all the stupid things you've done and to accept yourself for the wonderful and unique person that you are. Some people see themselves from the point of their flaws. Each of us is defined by our thoughts about ourselves, so we need to be careful not to allow ourselves to go on automatic. We are a sum total of our

---

[106] We die and are reborn each time we have a series of enlightening experiences or growth experiences because the person that we were changes as we grow and emerge as different people with different ideas. When old beliefs die, new ones emerge.

beliefs and our experiences, so make sure you want to be associated with your beliefs. This does not mean that we have to be limited by our experiences and beliefs or defined by them. If we do not take over and point our thoughts in the right direction, they can go in all different directions and drive a person haywire. Focus them on loving you and getting what you want.

Humans have a tendency to lean towards the negative if they allow their brains to run on automatic. However, we have evolved to the point where we know now that we can consciously take over and run our brains and decide which direction we want it to go in. And the people who know that, do it.

Remember the movie **Field Of Dreams**? Disasters were occurring in the middle of miracles. Life is like that. But what did the people in Field of Dreams do? They focused on the miracles, and greatly diminished the negative since they were doing the best they could about the situation. It's that simple: we have a choice between focusing on the negative or focusing on the positive, being happy and being unhappy only when we realize that we have it. Then we can choose happiness and bliss, and we'll have it. Sometimes, if it does not come naturally, you can make it happen with just a little rational arguing with yourself. Modifying negative feelings and thoughts is easier than you think.

Learned to conquer fear. Many people are living and running on fear and some of them do not even know it. Yet they are constantly fearful that things won't work out, that their jobs, relationships, friendships, won't work. Some carry a fear that they just don't quite measure up, or are not good enough. These kinds of fears can become subliminal and slip into the background, where they fester and can expand into every aspect of a person's life. They need to be routed out and eliminated. Sometimes, if they have been repressed, searching and routing them out can be difficult and painful, but well worth the effort. The Lifespring Basic Training is one place where you can dynamite away the 12-inch thick invisible wall of glass you have placed yourself inside in order to feel no pain. Do you feel like you're not really living? Have you lost the ability to feel? This training will make you live and feel again.

You have the ability to give your life not only meaning, but joy and bliss! Seek it! You can find it.

Make it a point to feed your soul once everyday.

Chapter 28

THE MOST
IMPORTANT
THINGS I DO THAT
KEEP ME YOUNG

Run or walk everyday at least 2 miles.

Eat at least 10 pieces of fruit a day, either as meals or as liquified fruit. Fruits and vegetables are natural medicines that contain tremendous healing substances. Foods can eliminate heart disease, high blood pressure, digestive disorders, fatigue, obesity and cancer.

Get a massage once a week to move body fluids that can get stuck. This process causes the entire body to become oxygenated. We have already learned how life- and health-giving oxygen is. When the body becomes fully oxygenated this acts as a switch that turns on the immune system, endorphins start to flow, stagnant fluids and toxins are moved. Consciousness becomes heightened. I am reborn balanced and whole again.

Take my vitamins, minerals, vitamin C, oxygen, kelp and amino acids. I have found that taking the proper amounts of these trace elements, especially B-complex and small amounts of amino acids two to three times a week creates a feeling of bliss and well-being in me. They also enhance color perception and flood me with a special new world of color and vibrancy. As long as I take the proper amounts of vitamins and minerals, eat well, exercise, grow and remain positive, I live in a virtual state of ecstasy and contentment.

Use Retin-A and exfoliants.

Do stretching for at least five minutes a day.

Use homeopathic remedies to heal myself. They have <u>no</u> side effects and work every time when properly prescribed and also stimulate the immune system, and thus, health!

Keep my mind wide open for any possibility. I do something to expand my mind everyday, even if it is only reading the newspaper.

Treat my life as the wonderful, precious gift that it is. Be grateful that my mother did not abort me. Rejoice in my health, in being in my right mind and perfectly formed. Rejoice in *ahimsa*, the doctrine that all life is sacred.

Chapter 29

```
HOW TO ELIMINATE THE
PAIN THAT MILLIONS
SUFFER IN SILENCE
```

Some of the things that can add years to your life for sure are peace, serenity and freedom from pain. Unfortunately, one half of all Americans are frantic 50 percent of the time, men, women and children included. This stress that we live with manifests itself in our bodies as pain.

The frantic progression of our lives has a lot to do with our stress. The parents are frantic and the kids assimilate it. Also the parents put heavy duty pressure on the kids to achieve, which increases their stress and eggs them into a frantic state. Increasingly, young people are committing suicide in response to this pressure. Where do we draw the line? We pressure our kids to do well because everyone wants the best for their kids. There has to be a better way than the way we've been doing it.

Why are we so frantic? Maybe it is because if we stop and look too closely at our lives we won't like what we see. We may find ourselves boring. So we keep on the move, telling ourselves, I have a busy life, so I must be interesting and not boring. Keeping busy can be a way of keeping things hidden, even from ourselves. We even hide upsets from ourselves, otherwise, why would we explode over anything? If things are rationally thought out first, rarely does an explosion occur. Life's little stresses and frantic and aggravating moments can also erupt every now and then in the form of back and neck pain.

Millions suffer these pains everyday of their lives. Office workers are especially vulnerable since they often sit for hours in one position causing their body fluids to clog up and get stuck in places. This manifests itself as stiff neck, shoulders or back. Added to this problem are the tensions that emerge among people working in offices. The seemingly simple but endless conflicts, if not resolved, can cause workers to be constantly tense, which blocks the flow of bodily fluids. If conflicts are not resolved, people often carry the tension around, which can become so painful as to even become life threatening.

I have actually had people come in to my clinic with frozen shoulders (some of which were cured in one visit), debilitating stiff necks, stiff from where the person has been working in an emotionally constricted environment and cannot relax their body. This tension and anxiety manifests itself as knots in the body, which are usually caused when their lymph fluid's flow is constricted by tension in the body.

Something that will contribute to your health and healing will be massage, which can eliminate most pains like magic and move stuck lymph fluids, mucous and congestion. A particularly effective massage is acupressure, which uses the acupuncture points to conduct electrical energy through meridians in the body and massively heal it. This fills the body with a sense of ecstasy because it becomes filled with endorphins which heal and start the chain of events that gets the immune system functioning fully, thus beginning the massive housecleaning of the body.

What Is Acupressure?

The Chinese discovered acupressure more than 5,000 years ago. They learned that pressing on certain points not only eliminated pain and tension but also helped other parts of the body. They discovered that pressure also benefitted the organs and immune system functioning.

Acupressure is an ancient way of healing that uses the fingers, knuckles and elbows to stimulate the body to heal itself. The process massively increases healing oxygen in the body and moves stuck fluids that can become putrid and painful. Acupressure is different from acupuncture in that acupuncture was discovered a few thousand years after acupressure, and acupuncture uses needles. Both use the same acupuncture points.

Acupressure is felt to be the most effective method for release of tension and stress and it is safe and natural.

There are special points of the body that conduct bioelectrical energy, what the Chinese have traditionally called "chi" and the Japanese call "ki" in which flows our life-force. When the points are pressed, toxins are moved into the blood, blood pressure is lowered and a natural high is experienced. Acupressure has been described as closing the gates to pain because it inhibits the pain signals sent to the brain. All these processes strengthen the body, promote health and increase resistance to disease. Acupressure also helps to re-balance the body and is equivalent to exercise. A one hour acupressure massage oxygenates the body as much as jogging for two miles at the same time that it strengthens the immune system, balances, lowers blood pressure, promotes healing and tranquility and induces a feeling of ecstasy.

If there is undue stress, then people have a tendency to tense up certain parts of their bodies, like the neck, or shoulders. When we sit for long periods on a regular basis (as office workers do), lymph and other fluids become blocked from the tension in the body and the inactivity. It is not long before the pain begins. There is a simple, natural acupressure procedure that will move stuck fluids and allow relief of the pain.

Right at the base of the skull on each side are two acupuncture points. Feel for them. You may feel swelling or knots that you never knew were there. Often pressing on these points will relieve a severe headache in five minutes.

Below those points on the tops of your shoulders right in the center of each one are two more points that become sore. Apply pressure with your fingers or a blunt object until you feel the relief. Also in the back, right under the tip of the wing of your shoulder blade are two points where fluids get stuck. Maneuver yourself in a way that you can apply pressure to them, or get a friend to help you by pressing on them. Press on the points for from two to ten minutes and you will be amazed at how much relief, clarity of mind and energy it brings.

To relieve the conflict, I recommend the Lifespring Basic Awareness Training for the feuding parties. They will return to work with the conflict resolved, and everyone else in the office will work a lot easier.

If you are having back or neck pain, pressing on the acupuncture point in the general area of the pain will often relieve it. Since stress generally collects in the acupuncture points of our bodies one of the secrets of relieving this pain is to relieve the stress in the points.

The procedure for doing acupressure is simple. Place the hands, knuckles, elbows, knees or fingers gently but firmly on the acupuncture points. You will get to know them when you feel them. Press, alternating the pressure until relief is felt. Make sure you get adequate feedback to ensure that the pressure is right. Pressure can be applied from two to five minutes at a time, but no more than ten minutes in one area. Work to the point that the acupressure makes the person sigh with relief until they feel very sleepy or fall asleep.

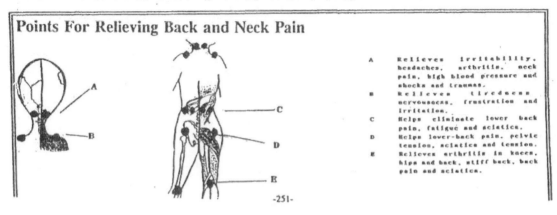

Points For Relieving Back and Neck Pain

A — Relieves irritability, headaches, arthritis, neck pain, high blood pressure and shocks and traumas.

B — Relieves tiredness, nervousness, frustration and irritation.

C — Helps eliminate lower back pain, fatigue and sciatica.

D — Helps lower-back pain, pelvic tension, sciatica and tension.

E — Relieves arthritis in knees, hips and back, stiff back, back pain and sciatica.

Chapter 30

A NATURAL CURE
FOR IMPOTENCE
AND MENSTRUAL
PROBLEMS

During my tenure as an acupressure practitioner, I have met hundreds of men who were impotent. Every one of them reported positive results with the acupressure treatment I used. A vitamin and mineral pill a day is helpful. The most important supplements to fight impotence are oxygen, L-Arginine, vitamin C, vitamin E, zinc and a mega vitamin and mineral every day. Many experienced complete relief after the first acupressure treatment. Many wives have called to thank me. Fortunately, the acupuncture points for curing impotence are the same as for curing menstrual problems. In addition, menstrual problems become virtually nonexistent if a woman does aerobic exercises for twenty minutes three times a week in most cases.

Impotence occurs sometimes as a result of anxiety, guilt about sex, pain in other parts of the body, high cholesterol, drugs, rigid religious teachings and emotional distress. Sometimes plain fear of not performing properly will lead to impotence. Chinese medicine believes that sexual activity is governed by the kidneys. Alcohol, caffeine, drugs, white sugar and flour all put a burden on the kidneys. Emotional duress puts a strain on the kidneys and it is advised that you seek out and eliminate yours. Talk to someone about it. The Chinese use beans to strengthen the reproductive organs. After 20 years of practicing acupressure, I have found all these things to be helpful.

Menstrual problems are usually caused by hormonal imbalances, which can be caused by diet and environmental pollution. Make sure you do not have a vaginal infection, since this can also be a cause. Another cause of menstrual problems is constipation or inflammation of the uterus or a contracted cervix.

Acupressure will re-regulate the endocrine system and stabilize hormonal imbalances, and thus, your emotions.

It has only been within the last few years that researchers discovered that the penis is a vascular organ. Therefore things that clog arteries like cholesterol and dietary fat affect blood flow to the penis. Smoking constricts blood vessels so you don't want to do that. Just two cigarettes a day prevent erections in test animals. Avoid stimulants like caffeine since they constrict the muscle that must dilate in order for an erection to occur.

If you have pain in your body, opiates that the body makes to relieve the pain turn off sexual feelings.

In addition to acupressure, taking a good vitamin and mineral supplement, B-complex, amino acids and oxygen will help alleviate both impotence and menstrual problems. All the systems in the body, the cardiovascular system, the endocrine system, the nervous system are vitally dependent on nutrition for proper functioning.

There are parts of the body that take precedence over others in getting nourishment when there is a deficiency. The brain gets priority, next are the heart and respiratory system. The first thing that gets neglected when there is a deficiency is sexual functioning, for it is low on the body's priority list.

Reduce proteins and eat more carbohydrates to increase libido. Some women who have had an IUD or used the pill lose interest in sex or have an inability to reach orgasm. The cause for this is most often organic. It could be a case of excessive estrogen or copper. To counteract this problem, eat foods rich in vitamins A, C and E and consume the minerals zinc and magnesium. Manganese has also proved to stimulate sexual desire. Many people experience an increase in sexual desire only days after beginning to take it. Thirty to fifty milligrams are adequate.

Vitamin A is extremely important to the production of the sex hormones. It keeps estrogen and progesterone balanced. Vitamin E is a detoxifier that has proved to stimulate libido. In fact, vitamin E deficiency is linked to lack of orgasm since it is mandatory for normal reflexes and for normal brain function. Both must be working properly for normal arousal. Magnesium has also been shown to play a part in sexual arousal. Look around you at the people you know.

People who are sexually satiated are far less aggressive than those who are sexually frustrated. You won't have any problem telling which is which.

Vitamin B$_6$ helps eliminate menstrual cramps and the effects of the pill. It also helps make women fertile. Phosphorus, a hormonal nutrient, is also a stimulator of libido. Sunshine has been proved to stimulate libido.

For many years we have known that the thyroid, which regulates metabolism, also influences sexual function. Potatoes are an iron-rich food that contain iodine, which the thyroid needs to keep healthy. For years a myth has existed that potatoes and starches like breads cause weight gain. Yet studies find that people who eat nutritious breads lose weight as a result of their bread intake alone. Example, two groups were given identical diets, except one group ate two slices of nutritious bread. They lost an average of 14 pounds over a two month period. The other group's weights remained constant or rose.

People suffering from impotence were given vitamin A and L-Arginine in separate studies and they experienced remarkable recoveries. Iodine is important for the production of hormones and is sometimes lacking in our diet. You need 150 micrograms a day.

Scientists have discovered that nitric oxide strongly influences erection and probably by the time you read this, you will be able to buy a nitric oxide preparation that will eliminate your impotence. Nitric oxide also works to stimulate libido in women. In the meantime, you can relieve impotence by using acupressure. An article in **The Washington Post** declares:

Nitric Oxide Signal Causes Erection, Scientists Discover

"We know of drugs that can generate nitric oxide and presumably elicit erection..."[107]

It used to be believed that only women have multiple orgasms, but a group of men have emerged who claim to be having them. They say a man's state of mind, and his believing that it is okay to have them will free him up to allow him

---

[107]   © 1993 **The Washington Post** by Boyce Rensberger, Reprinted with permission.

to experience them. Many men experience non-ejaculatory orgasms without realizing it because they think an orgasm must elicit fluid, though that is not necessarily so. A new book tells how any man can have multiple orgasms. It is called **Any Man Can** by Hartman and Fithian. They say every man who has tried their technique has been successful.

To experience a super orgasm, there is a sexual position that will help you attain it. The male needs to be in the override position on top of the female so that his penis is inside her vagina and pressing right against her clitoris. This position must be maintained at all times.

The couple can stimulate themselves to the edge of ecstasy and then back off and build it back up again and again until they can no longer hold back. In this way, they can make the act last a lot longer, and each can attain many small orgasms before the final display. This builds up to an incredible electrifying orgasmic release. The most important thing to remember is that you two must learn to fall into a natural rhythm of movement while keeping the initial position.

The side effects reported after having such a strong intimate encounter are increased intimacy and more acceptance of the other person, along with closer bonding of the couple. Sexual intimacy can lead to love, although love should lead to sexual intimacy.

I found information in **The Better Sex Video Series**, which is a superb teaching tool, that will improve anyone's sexual experiences, no matter how satisfying or experienced they may be. To order call 1-800-888-1900.

Some drugs can hinder ejaculation but not orgasm, like Melaril (prescribed for depression/anxiety). Chronic prostrate infections can do the same.

Avoid taking Mevacor (lovastatin) as it has been found to cause muscle damage, weakness, cramps, elevation of muscle enzyme in blood, abnormal electromyograms, liver damage, GI problems, and possible kidney failure. It inhibits the body's production of coenzyme Q^{10}, which is made by the body along with cholesterol. Thus, Mevacor reduces the synthesis of cholesterol as well as coenzyme Q^{10}, which is known to be a critical determinant of cardiac function.[108]

The procedure for doing acupressure to eliminate impotence is simple and is repeated here. Simply place the hands, knuckles or fingers on the acupuncture points illustrated and press, alternating the pressure until relief is experienced. A soft kneading will loosen the fascia[109] and make eliminating knots and swollen and sore areas a lot easier.

Acupressure should feel like a relief. If it hurts, it is being done too deeply. Never press directly on bones. Never press on deteriorating discs or fractured, delicate or broken bones. Help the person you get to do the procedures described here find your pain so it can be eliminated. In some cases there is no pain, but swelling in the acupuncture points. Eliminating it can increase your ability to concentrate and solve problems, get you on a higher level of consciousness, increase vitality and life span and restore sexual function.

Pressure can be applied from two to five minutes at a time, but no more than ten minutes in one area. Any pain you experience should feel like a relief, and not actual pain.

Soreness is common, especially if an area is tender when the work begins. As a rule, the soreness results from the swelling in the area, which distends the tissues and causes pain. Acupressure releases the swelling, the toxins go into the blood, and it takes a day or two for the tissues to return to normal.

Following are the acupuncture points that relieve impotency and menstrual problems. As I said I have never worked on an impotent male that this therapy did not help! The same is true for menstrual problems. Everyone I treated with acupressure for these problems reported positive results.

Grab a wife, friend, girlfriend, boyfriend and get rid of impotence and menstrual problems using acupressure!

Having menstrual cramps? They are caused by congealed blood. Bounce, walk, go shopping, and they will go away.

---

[108]   © 1993 by Life Extension Foundation, PO Box 229120, Hollywood, FL 33022-9120. 1-800-841-LIFE. Reprinted with permission.

[109]   Fascia is the fibrous connective tissue forming sheets or layers beneath the skin for enclosing muscles or internal organs.

Points For Relieving Impotency And PMS

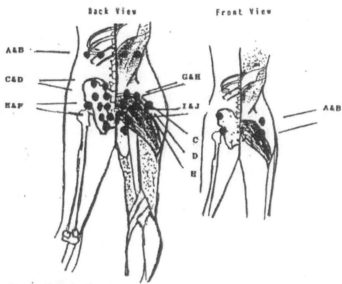

Back View   Front View

Points For Relieving Impotency

A&B Relieves impotency, premature ejaculation, reproductive problems, low back pain.

C&D Relieves sexual/reproductive problems, retention of urine, hip pain.

E&F Relieves impotency, sacral and sciatic pain.

G&H Relieves impotency and lumbago.

I&J Relieves vaginal discharge, genital pain, sterility.

K&L Relieves impotency, menstrual distress

M Relieves impotency, reproductive problems, irregular periods, urinary problems.

N Called the Three Mile Point, stimulation strengthens the entire body and helps the sexual reproductive system. It could take months, but stimulating this point will relieve impotence.

O Strengthens reproductive system, relieves impotency, vaginal discharge.

P Relieve impotency, vaginal discharge, strengthens reproductive system.

Points For Relieving PMS

A&B will usually relieve menstrual pain.

C Relieves cramping, painful hip, urine retention, problems related to reproduction.

D Relieves impotency, sterility, genital pain and painful sciatic.

E These points, called the sacrum, relax the uterus and relieve cramps.

To relieve the symptoms of menopause, supplement your diet with sesame seeds three times a week. Eat alfalfa, anise, apples, barley, carrots, cherries, fennel, garlic, hops, oats, parsley, potatoes, red beans, soybeans. These foods along with vitamins E and B6 can alleviate the depression, hot flashes, fatigue, loss of interest in sex and emotional instability that come with menopause.

Make sure you get enough calcium, magnesium and B_6. They work best when taken with the foods described above.

Exercise is important in every aspect of your life, and it can really ease menopause. A study of sedentary men found that one of the most significant changes was in their sex drive: they were one third more active. They also reported that they had more orgasms and fewer incidents of impotence. Sexual arousal and orgasm came easier as well. Women were affected the same as men.

One of the big dangers of the postmenopausal years is osteoporosis. Exercise along with diet and balanced supplements are the best measures to take for maintaining bone density and strength, especially of the immune system.

To give you an example of this in action: I have been exercising and eating hormone rich foods for twenty-five years, and my younger sister, who has not, is going through menopause, while my body has not even thought about it yet! I act, feel and look like I'm twenty. I am thinking about having a baby! I have discovered that how I think and <u>feel</u> about all this is most important of all. Yes, I imagine that I am 20 years old.

There is a group in California which advocates that people can be immortal. I totally embrace this concept because only when people believe things like this can they come true. There was a time when it was thought that cells could not regenerate. Yet, in philosophy, the concept comes up over and over: that beliefs have everything to do with what can and cannot be accomplished. People believed they could go to the moon, and they did. People who did not believe it did not. Only people who believe they can do something will accomplish it. Anyone who thinks he can't be president won't, and only one who believes he can will become president. People who believed they could develop a skin cream that would remove the top layer of skin and leave behind new baby skin developed it! Look at the power of beliefs!

Information is powerful. It can change your life.

Chapter 31

A NATURAL CURE
FOR MIGRAINE OR
ANY HEADACHE

Most headaches are caused by emotions, tension and dehydration. I believe that 90 percent of all headaches are a result of dehydration. They can be a signal that the brain is not getting enough oxygen. If any of the vertebrae of the neck are not in alignment, a headache can result. They are also caused by a misaligned cervix or constipation. In most cases, two or three glasses of water should relieve a headache after about ten minutes. I have used acupressure in dozens of cases to relieve migraines. In almost every case, I have used acupressure to eliminate 5- to 3-day old headaches in five minutes. The most it has ever taken has been fifteen minutes.

Many of my patients were introduced to me through someone who had come to me for migraine relief. Headaches, and especially migraines, can be caused by the body having to process an overload of toxins and the resultant overload causes the liver to produce the headache as an indication that the body needs fluids. I have discovered that if I maintain my fluid intake, I never get a headache.

Notice that when you get a migraine, it occurs after you have gone for a prolonged period without a sufficient amount of fluids. For example one busy day in the office, I did not get a chance to drink all day. I kept meaning too, but things kept happening one after the other, and by lunchtime, I had a splitting headache, the kind that left me totally helpless. Add to the fact that I had run at 5:30 in the morning and an unexpected phone call threw me late in my routine, and I did not have my traditional breakfast, and thus, the fluids I needed to prevent the headache. I could barely drive myself home and get to bed.

So notice when you start to get any headache, and there are all kinds, that you have gone for too long without fluids. If you work in an office environment and get frequent headaches, notify your superiors in advance of your condition and ask for permission to take fifteen or so minutes to relieve your headaches when they come. Having a time out to relieve your headache, and the relief of knowing that you will not have to suffer through it will be a big relief for you. It will increase your productivity at work, for you won't be sitting there for hours suffering with a headache and trying to be productive at the same time that you are waiting for what you took for the headache to get rid of it.

Relieve the headache while it is still a small headache, preferably, as soon as you become aware of it beginning. First drink at least two ten ounce glasses of water. If all you have is coke or chocolate milk, drink that. Some fluids are better than none. Go into a quiet room and use the techniques described below to relieve your headache. Deep breathing or meditating is recommended while you work on your acupuncture points.

Back in the early days when a migraine hit me (starting as a teenager), I had to go to bed. Aspirin, prescription drugs, herb teas, I tried everything, but, nothing helped until I discovered drinking water and acupressure. I learned to get rid of the headache when it was small as soon as it started by drinking so that it did not turn into a big headache and using acupressure. You must learn this as well and you will be headache free. Headaches and migraines can disappear from your life.

Work on the acupuncture points illustrated. A migraine should take five minutes to relieve if the right pressure is being used. A terrible migraine might take ten or fifteen minutes to relieve. The keys to relief are quiet, fluids, no stress and proper pressure on the acupuncture points.

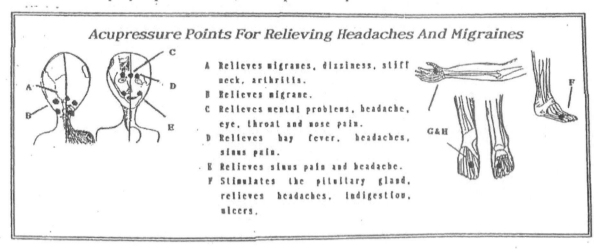

Acupressure Points For Relieving Headaches And Migraines

A Relieves migranes, dizziness, stiff neck, arthritis.
B Relieves migrane.
C Relieves mental problems, headache, eye, throat and nose pain.
D Relieves hay fever, headaches, sinus pain.
E Relieves sinus pain and headache.
F Stimulates the pituitary gland, relieves headaches, indigestion, ulcers.

Large amounts of vitamin C (250-1,000 mg/day) relieves headaches and. in some cases. asthma. This varies per individual.[110]

But taking vitamin C and then stopping can cause headaches. Therefore, make your vitamin C intake a bit consistent.

A good daily dosage is 250-1,000 mg/day. But in cases of illness, 250 mg or 500 mg every two or three hours for two or three days has proved helpful in fighting off infections. Do not take large doses of vitamin C for long periods of time especially if you notice that you get a smell of ammonia in your face, or coming from your body. Drink plenty of water and alkaline fluids and cut back on your dosage.

I read that vitamin C worked wonders against migraines and asthma. I casually mentioned to a mother who had a nine year old child with severe asthma and to an asthma sufferer that I had read a new study claiming this.

I discovered two months later that both had taken what I said to heart. When I saw the mother again she reported that she was no longer taking off from work for her child's asthma as she had been before she started her child on vitamin C before bed. She said her child reported that now she could play on the playground whereas she had previously had to sit and watch because of her asthma. This mother could not thank me enough.

When I saw the asthma sufferer again, she was not huffing and puffing as usual. She said she had gone out and bought some esterified vitamin C and that her asthma had greatly improved although she had been doubtful that it would help. She was very grateful that I told her about the study.

---

[110]   I tried taking 2,000 mg. per day after reading Linus Pauling's theories that our diets were once similar to that of monkeys so we need 2-6,000 mg. of vitamin C per day. On 2,000 mg. of vitamin C I had a bad reaction.

NOW! *Freely Available To Americans...*
EUROPEAN SMART DRUGS!

You don't have to wait for the FDA to "approve" of new memory and intelligence enhancing therapies. For your personal use, you can obtain therapies that can:

- Enhance mental function *four times* better than Hydergine!
- Increase mental energy, concentration, and alertness!
- Maximize the ability to memorize facts, figures, and scientific findings!
- Increase learning, mental agility, and I.Q.
- Improve test scores leading to higher grades and work productivity
- Prevent and treat degenerative brain diseases including Alzheimer's Disease, Parkinson's Disease, etc.

The Life Extension Foundation has compiled the sources, the doctors and the information to enable Americans to obtain life extension drugs from around the world. These drugs have been safely used in France, Germany and other countries for years, but until now, have been denied to Americans.

Europeans are using these drugs to improve their mental condition to unprecedented levels. Now Americans can gain access to advanced life extension therapies such as Piracetam, Centrophenoxine, human growth hormone, and a new memory-enhancing product that is *four times* more effective than Hydergine.

As a member of The Life Extension Foundation, you will learn about the scientific basis for using these life-enhancing therapies, their side effects, and how you can get them!

For just $50.00, you will receive *Life Extension Report* and *Life Extension Update* each month plus:

1. *The Directory Of Life Extension Doctors.* A nationwide directory of doctors who are knowledgeable about these advanced therapies and may be willing to prescribe them for you.

2. *The Physician's Guide To Life Extension Drugs.* The first book ever published to provide American doctors with information about safe and effective "unapproved drugs". This book is referenced to enable the lay person to understand and find therapies for specific purposes.

3. *The Directory Of Innovative Medical Clinics.* If you were told you had an incurable disease would you believe your doctor? A disease your doctor says is "untreatable" may already have a cure that the FDA has not yet "approved" of. There are scientists with impeccable credentials who are effectively treating so-called "terminal" victims of cancer, Alzheimer's Disease, etc. You can now access these advanced research centers with *The Directory Of Innovative Medical Clinics.*

4. *Discounts of 25% to 50%* on your vitamin purchases. Members buy name brand nutrient supplements and advanced life extension formulas at super discount prices.

5. *Discounts of 20%* on all your prescription drug purchases including popular life extension drugs such as Hydergine and Eldepryl. THE MAIL-ORDER PHARMACY saves members hundreds of dollars a year on their prescription drug purchases.

The Life Extension Foundation is the *only* organization in the world that tells you how to obtain the most advanced life extension therapies in the world...long *before* they are "approved" by the FDA. You will be the *first* to find out about products that will enhance your life

To join, use the coupon or call: 1-800-678-8989

Enclosed is my $50.00 membership. Please enroll me in your life extension program which includes two newsletters each month and the three directories of life extension doctors, drugs, and clinics and the super discounts on my vitamin and prescription drug purchases.

Mail to:
Life Extension Foundation
P.O. Box 229120
Hollywood, FL 33022

Name_____

Address_____

City _____ State _____ Zip_____

Credit Card # _____ Exp Date _____

Chapter 32

GRANTS, SCHOLARSHIPS AND CO-OP EDUCATION COULD MAKE YOUR DREAMS COME TRUE

Not many people know it but every year BILLIONS of dollars in scholarship, grant and endowment funds go unclaimed. If people don't know the money is out there, they don't go looking for it. I remember when I got out of high school, I knew I knew everything. It was only after my first year of college that I realized how much I did not know.

Getting an education has been one of the single most valuable experiences of my life, and to this day, I continue my education. However, I think of how impossible college once seemed to me, and how, if I had not found out, by sheer accident, about the billions of dollars worth of grant and scholarship money that goes unclaimed every year, I never would have gotten my education. I often wonder what would have become of me.

Co-op education is an attractive way to get an education if you have limited funds. Talk to your high school or college adviser about it. Some students are terrified about the counselor knowing about their financial situation or other personal things about their family. Forget this way of thinking and let it go. Instead, think of how you could be letting this thought stand in the way of an opportunity for a better life.

Statistics report that high school dropouts actually make less and less each year, whereas college graduates salaries are constantly on an upscale move. Which category do you want to be in?

Usually co-op education works like this: your college counselor sets up an interview with a Fortune 500 company for you. If they like you, they subsidize your education, you pay less tuition, you get to work part-time at the company to get practical information and valuable job training while you're in school. At the end of two to four years, you get your degree! And you have valuable job training with a large company that will probably hire you full-time and promote you after you get your degree.

Economics affect the quality of life. If you are working a minimum wage job because you never had a chance to start or finish a degree, there are a number of ways that you can start or finish your degree, from cooperative education programs to Saturday college, night school, numerous scholarships and fellowships available due to your religious or other past or present affiliations. You can even benefit from your parents' past or present affiliations. For example, there is a scholarship fund for children of veterans, Catholics, Protestants. There are now available billions of unclaimed dollars sitting in these funds waiting to be picked up. Take a look at the Student Data Form. All those classifications have awards available.

There are colleges and institutions all over the country that are free, like the Parsons School in New York and The Milton Hershey School for adolescents in Hershey, PA. In Washington, DC there is the free Washington Saturday College (202-581-9176 or 202-723-4648. Seek and you will find them.

Keep in mind that health benefits being granted to 37 million uninsured Americans is going to make the demand for doctors and their salaries go through the roof. That might be a good career choice for you. You get respect, dignity and paid what you are worth.

An article in The New York Times talked about cheaper federal student loans at 105 colleges.

"When a student applies for a direct loan, the college will electronically send the application to the Education Department, which will decide within 72 hours and send a check."[111]

Colleges and the funds and organizations that have the money never advertise these opportunities. But all you have to do is ask. My mother used to say your

---

[111]   © **1993 The New York Times Company.**

mouth is made to open it and ask for what you want. When I do I get what I ask for. Try this in all aspects of your life. You will be amazed at the results!

Back to getting in school, simply ask at the school you are interested in about their financial aid, scholarship and grant programs and most importantly, their cooperative education programs. This important program allows the student to work at the school, the school places the student in a position, usually with a Fortune 500 company, and the student receives a degree at the end of three or four years, sometimes less, for one third of the cost of a college degree.

If you have a child that is giving you trouble, a good cure is a geographical one. Check the **Peterson's Guides** for a school that offers a guaranteed tuition plan, which usually means that grants are available, or the student can work at the school to earn his tuition.

The **Directory of Financial Aids For Minorities** and **Lovejoy's** college guides list thousands of sources of little-known grants and scholarships that are available.

Federally Supported Financial Aid Programs are: Pell Grants where from 1,000-3,000 dollars per year are granted to the student; the National Direct Student Loan Program; the Educational Opportunity Grant Program where the student is awarded a grant of 1,000-1,500 dollars per year; the College Work-Study Program, where the student pays off part or all of his educational expenses by working part-time at the school; and the Guaranteed Student Loan Program where a student may borrow from a bank, credit union or savings institution and the State or other agency guarantees the loan usually with an interest rate far below traditional rates. Interest starts accruing after you graduate from college.

Another is the Educational Opportunity Grants Program (BEOG and SEOG) which is usually a grant of 1,000 per year for four years.

Pell grants are available and do not have to be repaid.

There are schools that have a guaranteed tuition plan. You can find them in the **Peterson's Guides**.

The United States offers Federal government money for thousands of Americans to get an education. The Reserve Officers Training Corps (ROTC). The ROTC Vitalization Act of 1964 authorized two ROTC programs for the Air Force. There are two and four year programs. For more information and to find out which schools offer the programs write:

Department of the Army
ROTC Directorate
Fort Monroe, VA 23351

Chief of Navy Personnel (Pers-B641)
Department of the Navy
Washington, DC 20370

Air Force ROTC
Office of Information
Maxwell Air Force Base, Alabama 36112

There are also:

The United States Military Academy at West Point

The United States Naval Academy at Annapolis

The United States Air Force Academy at Colorado Springs

These are all by appointment and involve competitive exams for admission.

Admission to The United States Coast Guard Academy at New London and The United States Merchant Marine Academy at Kings Point is on the basis of competitive exams after authority to take them is given.

There is the National Direct Student Loan Program where the student may borrow 2,500-5,000 dollars per year for college costs and pay the money back at a low interest rate after school is finished.

Tuition At Campus Is Free
For All Black Freshmen

"Florida Atlantic University this fall will offer free tuition to every black freshman who meets admission standards, school officials said."[112]

For more information on how to obtain funding, contact:

National College Scholarship Foundation
600 S. Frederick Avenue, 2nd Floor
Gaithersburg, MD 20877

Dan Case
National Scholarship Research Service
PO Box 2516
San Rafael, CA 94912

Off To College
PO Box 361
Cardiff, CA 92107

Guide To Programs
US Government Printing Office
Washington, DC 20550

---

[112]   Reprinted with permission of The New York Times, New York, NY 3/9/90.

SOURCES OF ALTERNATIVE HEALTHCARE:

American Association of Naturopathic Physicians
2366 Eastlake Avenue E. Suite 323
Seattle Washington   phone 206-323-7610

American Association of Naturopathic Physicians
their local number from the Washington DC Metropolitan area 202-244-1978

American Institute For Homeopathy
1585 Glencoe
Denver Colorado 90220

Center For Science In The Public Interest, 1875 Connecticut Avenue NW, Suite 300, Washington, DC
20009

Homeopathic Educational Services
2036 Blake
Berkeley California 94704. The largest homeopathic resource store with books and tapes available by
mail or phone 510-649-0294

Hospital Santa Monica
738 Design Court Suite 301
Chula Vista California 91911 phone 1-800-359-6547

International Bio-Oxidative Medicine Foundation
PO Box 13205
Oklahoma City Oklahoma 73112-1205 phone 405-478-4266(IBOM)

International Foundation For Homeopathy
2366 Eastlake Avenue
Seattle Washington 98105

Longevity Magazine
1965 Broadway
New York New York 10023

National Center For Homeopathy
801 North Fairfax Suite 306
Alexandria Virginia 22314

National Health Federation
PO Box 688
Monrovia California 91017

Successful Aids Treatments (a 20-page research paper on alternative therapy for AIDS) 1-800-284-6263

The Family News (an alternative health newspaper)
9845 NE 2 Avenue
Miami Shores Florida 33138 phone 1-800-284-6263

The Life Extension Foundation
2490 Griffin Road
Fort Lauderdale Florida 33312 phone 1-800-841-5433

Well Mind Society Of Greater Washington
1141 Georgia Avenue
Silver Spring Maryland 20910 phone 301-949-8282

REFERENCES:

2 Admit EPA Violated Hazardous Waste Law In Issuing Permit. The New York Times 1992

2 Women At Rocky Flats Plant Tell Of Intimidation, Safety Violations. The Washington Post 1991

2,400 Beach Closings Tied to Old Sewers, A Study Says, The New York Times, 8-15-91

Acne Drug Side Effect; New Age In Skin Care? Wrinkles, Sun Damage Reversed, The Washington Post, 1-22-88

After Years Of Skepticism, Vitamins Win Support As Agents Of Health, The New York Times, 1991

Agency Cites Urgent Need To Fight Increase In TB. The New York Times 1992

Alkaline Hydrogen Peroxide Unlocks Energy In High-Fiber Lignified By-Products, 252 Nutrition Reviews, Vol 44, No7/7-86

Alternative Medicine Yellow Pages, The Life Extension Foundation 1-800-544-4440

American Association Of Naturopathic Physicians, 2366 Eastlake Avenue E. #323, Seattle, WA 98102 phone 206-323-7610. In the DC metropolitan area phone 202-244-1978

American Institute For Homeopathy, 1585 Glencoe, Denver, CO 90220

An Epidemic In Disguise, by Sherry Baker, Omni Magazine, 1965 Broadway, New York, NY 3-88

Anger Lingers After Leak At Atomic Site. The New York Times 1992

Ann Landers on Herpes, The Washington Post 7-2-90

Appeals Court Strikes Down OSHA Standards On Toxic Exposure, The Washington Post 1992

Bethesda Co-Op, 6500 Seven Locks Road, Cabin John, MD

Bethesda Crisis Center, 4910 Auburn Avenue, Bethesda, MD 20814. 301-656-9161.

Birth And Bacteria, USA Today, PO Box 500, Washington, DC, 10-13-88, Lifeline

Boundary Waters, PO Box 26173, Minneapolis, MN 55426, phone 612-823-9236

Break In Pipe Spews Sewage Near San Diego's Shore, The New York Times 1992

Can Exercise Fight The Effects Of Aging? The New York Times, 1991

Center For Science In The Public Interest

Chemicals That Taint Seafood, The Washington Post 1992

Chemists Learn Why Vegetables Are Good For You, The New York Times, 1993

Chemists Learn Why Vegetables In Diet Help People Avoid Cancer, The New York Times, 1990

Childbed Fever And Hand Washing. The Washington Post 1992

Committed Interaction, by Ann P. Miller, Lifespring Bulletin, Winter 1988

Cosmopolitan, 224 W. 57 St, New York, NY 10019

Court Affirms Ban On Carcinogenic Pesticides In Processed Foods, The Washington Post 1992

Creager's Human Anatomy and Physiology by Joan C. Creager. Wadsworth Publishing Company, Belmont, CA Curing Type A, The Trusting Heart by, Redford Williams, MD. Psychology Today, 24 E. 23 St, New York, NY. 1-2-89 pgs. 36-42

Cynicism and Mistrust Tied to Early Death, The New York Times, 1-17-89

Crystal Oxygen, AACHT. Product/Usage Briefing No. 89

Dangerous Hormone. The New York Times 1993.

Debris Calls Attention To Disposal of Med-Waste, The Birmingham News, 7-10-88

De-Stress Your Life, The Hope Heart Institute, 1988

De-Stress Yourself, The Washington Post, 1993

Detective Story, Brain Turns To Sponge And Scientists Find Some Bizarre Clues, The Wall Street Journal, 2-91

Discovering Homeopathy by Dana Ullman, published by North Atlantic Books, Berkeley CA 1991

Do Your Eyes Grow? The New York Times 1992.

Does Ozone Alleviate AIDS Diarrhea? Medical Hypotheses, Raven Press, Ltd., From the Rehabilitation Medicine Service, San Francisco Veterans Administration Medical Center (SFVAMC) and the Department of Orthopaedic Surgery, University of California, San Francisco School of Medicine (MTC...JMG) San Francisco, CA, USA 1993

Donsbach, Kurt W, M.D. 738 Design Court, Suite 301, Chula Vista, CA 91911 619-482-8533

E.P.A. Urged To Ease Rules On Cleanup Of Toxic Waste. The New York Times 1992

Eating Seafood? Put Safety First, Parade Magazine, 750 Third Avenue, New York, NY 9-11-88,

Eating Well, Is That Food Really Safe? The Washington Post 3-15-89

Economic Assistance Service, 9351 Bremerton Way, Gaithersburg, MD 20879

Estimates Of Weapons Cleanup Inflated. The New York Times 1992.

Everything You Ever Wanted To Know About Nutrition by David Reuben. Simon & Schuster, 1230 Avenue of the Americas, New York, NY 10020

Exercise, A Little Bit'll Do You, The Washington Post 1993

Exercise Is The Fountain Of Youth by Jane Brody, The New York Times, 1986

Experiments Suggest Brain Cells Regenerate. The Washington Post 1992

F.D.A. Warns Of Toxins In Some Crab Organs, The Washington Post 1992

Facing A Nightmare Of Poisoned Earth. The Washington Post 1991

Foods Are Cure For What Ails You, by Mary Evertz, The Washington Times, 3400 New York Avenue NE, Washington, DC 11-9-90

Forgiveness As Love, by Judith Hart, Sources, 4-5-88

Fortified Foods Could Fight Off Cancer, The New York Times, 1991

Fortified Foods Could Help Ward Off Cancer, The New York Times, 2-19-91

Fortune, Time & Life Building. Rockefeller Center, New York, NY 10020

G.A.O. Faults Regulators On Reproductive, Developmental Hazards, The New York Times, 1992

G.A.O. Urges Suspension Of New Pesticide Testing Program. The New York Times 1992

Garlic: It Gets In Your Blood, Center For Science In The Public Interest

Germs In The Chalice, The New York Times, 4-6-91

Good Fish...Bad Fish, Center For Science In the Public Interest, Washington, DC 10-88 cover story

GAO Faults Regulators On Reproductive, Developmental Hazards, by Michael Weisskopf, The Washington Post 10-2-91, pg. A4

Hand-Washing Practices A Problem In Hospitals. The Washington Post 1993

Hanford Cleanup Could Cost $57 Billion, The New York Times, 1-20-90

Hanford Site Cleanup Seen As Daunting Task. The Washington Post 1991

Harvard Medical School Health Letter and Mental Health Letter, 25 Shattuck Street, Boston, MA 02115

Healthtalk: Waking Up On Sleep, The Washington Post 3-30-84

Hearing-Loss Study Hints At Reviving Cells. The New York Times 1993

Heretical Theory On Brain Diseases Gains New Ground, The New York Times, 10-8-91, pg. C1

High Mercury Levels Found In Everglades Game Fish, The Washington Post

Homeopathic Educational Services, 2036 Blake, Berkeley, CA 94704. The largest homeopathic resource store with books and tapes available by mail or phone 510-649-0294

Hope Emerges As Key To Success In Life, The New York Times, 1992

Hospital Santa Monica, 738 Design Court #301, Chula Vista, CA 91911. 1-800-359-6547.

Hot Angelenos Gaze Longingly At Beaches' Forbidden Waves, The New York Times, 1992

How The Mind Heals, by Alan Anderson, Psychology Today, 12-82

How You See Yourself, Potential for Big Problems, The New York Times, 2-7-91

Hudson PCB Removal Stalled Again, The New York Times, 1-16-91, pg. B4

Human Nutrition by Scientific American. W. H. Freeman and Company, publishers

Hydrogen Peroxide, by Dr. Donsbach, pgs. 1-7, 10

International Bio-Oxidative Medicine Foundation, PO Box 13205, Oklahoma City, OK 73113-1205 phone 405-478-4266(IBOM)

International Foundation For Homeopathy, 2366 Eastlake Avenue, Seattle, WA 98105

Introduction To Mordern Existentialism by Ernst Breisach published by Grove Press, Inc., New York.

Lead In Greenland Is Traced To The U.S., The New York Times, 1993

Leaking Tanks Pose Risks, Raise Cleanup Costs For Area Residents. The Washington Post 1992.

Letter to Hospital Santa Monica from Debbie Silbernagel, who was cured of cancer there 10-22-89

Lifespring, 4650 East West Highway, Bethesda, MD 20814 (They have offices in most major cities)

Lifestyles Of The Healthy And Hearty, Redford Williams, MD, Psychology Today, 1/2-89 pg. 35

Longevity, 1965 Broadway, New York, NY 10023

Loss Of Iron Linked To Exercise, The Washington Post, 1993

Medical Debris Washes Up In Arundel, The Washington Post, 1990

Medical Hypotheses, Does Ozone Alleviate AIDS Diarrhea? Raven Press, Ltd., From the Rehabilitation Medicine Service, San Francisco Veterans Administration Medical Center (SFVAMC) and the Department of Orthopaedic Surgery, University of California, San Francisco School of Medicine (MTC...JMG) San Francisco, CA, USA

MEGA-NUTRITION FOR WOMEN by Richard A. Kunin, M.D. McGraw-Hill Book Company, New York, NY 1983.

Mind/Body Connection, NIH - 9000 Rockville Pike, Bethesda, MD 20982

Moderate Workouts Reduce Stress, Anxiety, Depression, The Washington Post, 1993

More Needles Wash Ashore in Arundel, The Washington Post 9-8-88

More Needles Wash Ashore in Arundel Contamination, The Washington Post 1988

Mosquito Is Linked To Deadly Virus, Worrying Health Officials. The Washington Post 1992

National Center For Homeopathy, 801 N. Fairfax, #306, Alexandria, VA 22314

National Institutes of Health, 9000 Wisconsin Avenue, Bethesda, MD

National Resources Defense Council

Newly Suspected Benefits Of Vitamins In The Body, The New York Times, 1992

New Pesticide Policy Leaves Residue of Questions, The Washington Post 10-24-88

Newsweek, 444 Madison Avenue, New York, NY 10022

Nitric Oxide Signal Causes Erection, Scientists Discover, The Washington Post 1992

No More Wrinkles? by Ann Giudici Fettner, Hippocrates, 301 Howard St. #1800, San Francisco, CA 94105. Jan/Feb 1988 pgs 20-22

Nuclear Waste Project Faltering Badly Under Civilian Safety Rule, The New York Times, 1-3-89

Nutritionists Look At Supplements As Weapons Against Chronic Illness, The Washington Post, 1993

Optimism Dims In Effort On Malaria As It Spreads, by Philip J. Hilts, The New York Times, 10-9-91

Organic...Or What? Bethesda Co-op News, 6700 Seven Locks Road, Cabin John, DC 4-91 pg. 2

Oxygen Therapies by Ed McCabe 1-800-284-6263

Parade Magazine, 750 Third Ave., New York, NY 10017

Pet-Borne Illnesses and Unsuspecting Owners, The Washington Post 7-17-90

Prescription For Nutritional Healing, by James & Phyllis Balch, Avery Publishing Group, 120 Old Broadway, Garden City Park, NJ

Prevention, 33 E. Minor St, Emmaus, PA 18090

Preventive Medicine, a Little Soap and Water, The Washington Post 9-25-85

Psychology Today, 24 E. 23rd Street, New York, NY 10010

Radiation Effect Played Down At Uranium Plant. The Washington Post 1991

Raven Press, Ltd., Does Ozone Alleviate AIDS Diarrhea from Medical Hypotheses, from the Rehabilitation Medicine Service, San Francisco Veterans Administration Medical Center (SFVAMC) and the Department of Orthopaedic Surgery, University of California, San Francisco School of Medicine (MTC...JMG) San Francisco, CA, USA, 1993

Replacement of Sand Planned At Copacabana, The New York Times

Report Looks To River Water To Fill New York City Needs, The New York Times

Report Ties Electrical Fields To Cancer, The New York Times, 12-15-90

Rise In Asthma Deaths Is Tied To Ignorance Of Many Physicians, The New York Times, 5-4-93

San Diego Lifts Quarantine On Some Beaches, The New York Times, 1992

Scholarship Funding Service, 10 Circuit Ct, Gaithersburg, MD 20878

Science, 1333 H St. NW, Washington, DC 20001

Self, 350 Madison Avenue, New York, NY 10017

Sewage Bacteria In Food Chain, The New York Times, 1993

Sharp Cut In Serious Birth Defect Is Tied to Vitamins In Pregnancy, The New York Times, 11-24-89

Should You Take Vitamins? by Stuart M. Berger, Parade Magazine, 750 3rd Avenue, New York, NY, 1989

Spill Is A Sign Of Wider Sewage Problems, The New York Times, 1992

Study Documents How Anger Can Impair Heart Function, The New York Times, 1992

Study Of Retail Fish Markets Finds Wide Contamination And Mislabeling, The New York Times, 1992

Study Finds Cream Clears Age Spots. The New York Times 1992

Stress May Be Something To Sneeze About, USA Today, 8-29-91, FP

Successful AIDS Treatments by Ed McCabe 1-800-284-6263

SUPERIMMUNITY by Paul Pearsall, Ph.D. McGraw-Hill Book Company, New York, NY 1987

TB, Easily Transmitted, Adds A Peril To Medicine. The New York Times 1992

Tank Leaks Pose Risk, Raise Costs. The Washington Post 1992

Telephone Reference, Montgomery County Library System, 301-217-4636

The American Association Of Naturopathic Physicians, 2366 Eastlake Avenue, Seattle, WA 98102, phone 206-323-7610. From the Washington, DC metropolitan area call 202-244-1978

The Aging Brain: The Mind Is Resilient, It's The Body That Fails, The New York Times, 1991

The Bacteria At The Table. The New York Times, 1990

The Better Sex Video Series, PO Box 5310, Lighthouse Point, FL 33074. 1-800-888-1900

The Complete Guide To Your Emotions And Your Health: New Dimensions in Mind/Body Healing by Emrika Padus and the Editors of Prevention. Mind & Medicine, Vol 1, No. 4

The Exercise RX, The Washington Post 3-5-90

The Family News, 9845 NE 2 Avenue, Miami Shores, FL 33138. 1-800-284-6263

The Life Extension Foundation, 2490 Griffin Road, Ft. Lauderdale, FL 33312 1-800-841-5433

The New York Times, 229 West 43 St, New York, NY 10036

The Oozing Of America, The Washington Post, 9-15-91

The Road Less Traveled by M. Scott Peck, Simon & Schuster, 1230 Ave of the Americas, New York, NY

The Washington Post, 1150 15th St. NW, Washington, DC 20071

The Secret Of Long Life? Be Dour And Dependable, The New York Times, 1991

The Awakened Life by Wayne Dyer from Nightingale Conant. A guaranteed winner. 1-800-525-9000
The Bacteria At The Table. The New York Times 5-8-90

Theory Links AIDS to Malaria Experiments, The New York Times 1991

Three Promising Weapons Against Disease, The New York Times, 9-25-91, pg. C11

Tighten The Rules On Seafood Safety, The New York Times, 1992

Top Scientists Warm Tuberculosis Could Become Major Threat. The New York Times 1992.

Top Worry: A Waste Tank That Belches. The Washington Post 1991

Toxic Agents Found To Be Killing Off Whales, The New York Times, 1992
Trade Pact Raises Threat Of TB From Cattle.

Unlimited Power, by Anthony Robbins. Ballantine Books, 1987

Uranium Dust At Ohio Plant Is Rated As High. The New York Times 1991

Viruses Central To Ocean Life, The Washington Post, 1991

Vitamin C Is Linked To Heart Benefit, The New York Times, 1992

Vitamin Pack Is Found To Aid Elderly, The New York Times, 1992

Vitamins Win Support As Potent Agents Of Health, The New York Times, 1991

Walking Found To Aid Heart, Regardless Of Pace, The New York Times, 1991

Washing Hands Can Be A Major Disease-Stopper--As Grandma Knew. The Washington Post 1985.

All ▾　barbara frank take 10 years off your face

Try Prime

Departments ▾　　Recommended For You

EN ▾ | Hello, Sign in
Account & Lists ▾　Orders　Try Prime ▾

Books　Advanced Search　New Releases　Amazon Charts　Best Sellers & More　The New York Times® Best Sellers　Children's Books　Textl

Stone & Beam　*Exclusively on Amazon*　　Shop now

‹ Return to product information　　Have one to sell?　　Every purchase on Amazon.com is protected by an A-to-z guarantee.　　Feedback on this p
you think

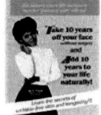

How to Take 10 Years Off Your Face Without Surgery and Add 10 Years to Naturally (Paperback)

by Barbara Frank (Author)

1 customer review　　Share

Price + Shipping	Condition (Learn more)	Delivery	Seller Information
$94.67 & FREE Shipping	**Used - Acceptable**	• Arrives between May 15-22.	**Thriftbooks**
$90.69 + $3.99 shipping	**Used - Very Good** Tight & Clean. No Marks. Light	• Arrives between May 15-22. • Want it delivered Thursday,	**sablevision** 94%
$179.21 & FREE Shipping	**Used - Acceptable** Cover appears used and pages	• Arrives between May 16-24. • Want it delivered Tuesday,	**Red Rhino** 91%
$179.33 & FREE Shipping	**Used - Good** Meets or exceeds Amazon	• Arrives between May 16-24. • Want it delivered Tuesday,	**Red Rhino** 91%
$230.57 & FREE Shipping	**Used - Very Good**	• Arrives between May 21-30. • Want it delivered Friday, May 25? Choose **Expedited**	**Chris's Bargains** 91%
$474.49 & FREE Shipping	**Used - Like New**	• Arrives between May 21-30. • Want it delivered Friday, May 25? Choose **Expedited**	Chris's Bargains 91%
$497.12 & FREE Shipping	**New**	• Arrives between May 21-30. • Want it delivered Friday, May 25? Choose **Expedited**	**Chris's Bargains** 91%
$1,184.10 & FREE Shipping	**New**	• Arrives between May 16-24. • Want it delivered Tuesday, May 22? Choose **Standard Shipping** at checkout. • Shipping rates and return policy.	**Red Rhino** 91% positive over the past 12 months. (7,272 total ratings)

Refine by Clear all

Shipping
☐ Free shipping
　☐ Very Good
　☐ Good
　☐ Acceptable

Testimonials:

I have experienced leg aches and backaches all of my life due to probably surgery at age 20 months. I wore a brace from ankle to head from age 20 months to age 6. At age 13-15 I also had surgery on my left knee which created more pain. The types of treatments that I have had are back surgery, epidural blocks, Acupuncture, Reike, Rolfing, Shiatsu, Hypnotism, Chinese Acupressure, and hundreds of massages to get rid of the pain. Everything was temporary, lasting usually less than 48 hours. Now I experience no leg aches and no back aches. Energy level has tripled. At age fifty, I have never felt any better physically. For the first time I can do manual labor without pain and I contribute this all to Barbara Frank's treatment and advice on general health and well being.

When I first came to Barbara, my hair was thinning and all white with a serious receding hairline. My hairline has improved, the hair in the back is very much back to original thickness and color. The receding hairline is moving forward instead of back. The hair is a bonus, but being without pain is unbelievable.

Terry

1 (443)-831-4112

I used my knee to move something and felt I hurt it. I came to you with my knee hurting me so badly. It was swollen and sore. For three days I suffered with it. It was swollen but it was fluid. I went to the hospital. They drew out the fluid. It was very painful to have the fluid drawn out and the next day it was back just as before and still very sore. The hospital said come back and we will do it again. Walking was very painful. At that point I turned to you, Barbara for help. Some of my friends who had had miracles performed had told me about you, but I did not believe them.

The pain went away after Barbara Frank worked on it. She told me what was causing the problem, gave me some herbs for it and my knee has been fine ever since. Without your help, it would have taken me months to heal.

Kofi

Ph. (703) 567-5164

April 1999

My name is Gloria T. Lancaster. I was injured in 1982 and had back surgery and knee surgery in 1990. I had terrible pain throughout my body and took medications for 18 years, Tylenol Four and Three were two of my prescriptions plus Soma, a muscle relaxant, which did not help me. I still felt the pain. My doctor told me, go home, there's nothing more I can do for you. I fell a lot. had tremors, vomiting, cramping in my legs as if I had muscular dystrophy. Everything I tried did not help. I had pain from my head to my toes, could barely talk or move, put on or take off my shoes. I could not do for myself, I had to be taken care of, so I moved to a Senior Citizens building for the disabled. Then I heard of Barbara Frank.

I heard of this woman through another friend, Andi. I took my chances and went to her knowing that nothing else helped me. My doctor had told me, go home, there's noting more I can do for you. I did not have the money for the treatment I needed but she was interested in the person, not just the money, and she allowed me to be treated. When I first went to her she gave me this wonderful vegetable juice which elevated me to a natural high. I could feel her spirit and tenacity from working with others and healing them. She informed me of the things that were wrong with my body and went to work on it, finding many other things wrong. She proceeded with the treatment. There was never anything like what she does. When she finished, after one session, I felt all my strength, felt completely normal, could tie my shoes, and even dance! It is a miracle!

(202) 332-6274

ABOUT MS. FRANK

The first printing of this book was done by one of Barbara's patients who came to her crippled after being in physical therapy for many years with little improvement. After two sessions with Barbara, he could walk straight, and without even reading her book, agreed to put it in book form. Ms. Frank started on the road to health when her daughter was born more than thirty years ago. The child was very sickly, and each prescription had an adverse effect on her. This lead Barbara to studying natural therapies. It was a blessing in disguise, for many have benefitted from what she has learned. The Institute of Chinese Culture (212-224-8880) on Grand Street in New York has made four television shows about her. She has been on Public Television on the tv show YOUR HEALTH IS YOUR WEALTH. She has been on radio more than a dozen times and speaks in front of groups and organizations. She is a Certified Lymphologist through The International Academy of Lymphology, and has studied many other natural healing modalities, including, The University of Maryland Alternative Medicine Intensive, Homeopathy, Herbal Therapy, Vitamin Therapy, Acupuncture, Acupressure, Shiatsu, Philosophy and Psychology as well as many consciousness-raising seminars like Lifespring Basic Awareness Training, John Grey Seminars, The Foundation For Peace Awareness Training, The Forum, Intuition Seminars and such.

December 9, 1994

Nobel Prize Committee

Nobel Foundation, Nobel House

Sturegatan 14

11436 Stockholm Sweden

I would like to join those who recommend Barbara Frank to be awarded with the forthcoming Nobel Prize for her new book: HOW TO TAKE 10 YEARS OFF YOUR FACE WITHOUT SURGERY AND ADD 10 YEARS TO YOUR LIFE NATURALLY.

This volume is unique, fulfilling spiritual and physical life, free of ailments, stresses, inhibitions.

The writer takes up the challenge of aging, a struggle which humans are destined to lose. "Not to give up, as long as we live"--that is her message. Her pulsating, dynamic style matches wonderfully the contents; the intentionally brisk sentences, short chapters are part of a well and logically organized structure, and enable her to deal with wide-ranging subjects, from college education for the poor to global pollution dangers to ways to overcome depression. She makes it clear, that her intention is to get this book accessible even to those who are less literate.

Put in the particular United States setting, the book gives hope and support to those who try to break the suffocating bonds of bleak circumstances, whether it is old age, a grave ailment, murderous addictions, like drugs and alcohol, or "just" life on the fringe of society. The writer herself treats gravely ill indigent patients free. Awarding her would be a recognition of all those who are dedicated to help their human brethren.

Please consider Ms. Barbara Frank for the prestigious award.

Richard Hirschler

Editor of Transition

The World Bank Newsletter

9 781884 994005